TRANSITION FROM
Clinician *to*
Educator
A PRACTICAL APPROACH

MARIA C. FRESSOLA, EdD, EdM, MA, RN, CNE
Professor of Nursing
Bergen Community College
Paramus, New Jersey

G. ELAINE PATTERSON, EdD, EdM, MA, APN, CNE
Professor of Nursing
Ramapo College of New Jersey
Mahwah, New Jersey

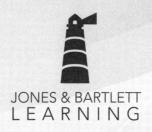

JONES & BARTLETT
LEARNING

World Headquarters
Jones & Bartlett Learning
5 Wall Street
Burlington, MA 01803
978-443-5000
info@jblearning.com
www.jblearning.com

Jones & Bartlett Learning books and products are available through most bookstores and online booksellers. To contact Jones & Bartlett Learning directly, call 800-832-0034, fax 978-443-8000, or visit our website, www.jblearning.com.

Substantial discounts on bulk quantities of Jones & Bartlett Learning publications are available to corporations, professional associations, and other qualified organizations. For details and specific discount information, contact the special sales department at Jones & Bartlett Learning via the above contact information or send an email to specialsales@jblearning.com.

Production Credits

VP, Executive Publisher: David D. Cella
Executive Editor: Amanda Martin
Acquisitions Editor: Teresa Reilly
Associate Editor: Danielle Bessette
Production Manager: Carolyn Rogers Pershouse
Associate Production Editor: Juna Abrams
Marketing Communications Manager: Katie Hennessy
Product Fulfillment Manager: Wendy Kilborn
Composition: S4Carlisle Publishing Services
Cover Design: Kristin E. Parker
Associate Director of Rights & Media: Joanna Lundeen
Rights & Media Specialist: Wes DeShano
Media Development Editor: Troy Liston
Cover Image: © mhlam/Shutterstock
Printing and Binding: Edwards Brothers Malloy
Cover Printing: Edwards Brothers Malloy

Library of Congress Cataloging-in-Publication Data
Names: Fressola, Maria C., author. | Patterson, G. Elaine, author.
Title: Transition from clinician to educator : a practical approach / Maria C. Fressola,
   G. Elaine Patterson.
Description: Burlington, Massachusetts : Jones & Bartlett Learning, [2017] |
   Includes bibliographical references and index.
Identifiers: LCCN 2016014953 | ISBN 9781284068740 (pbk.)
Subjects: | MESH: Education, Nursing—manpower | Faculty,
   Nursing—organization & administration | Nurse's Role—psychology
Classification: LCC RT62 | NLM WY 18 | DDC 610.73076—dc23
LC record available at https://lccn.loc.gov/2016014953

6048

Printed in the United States of America
20 19 18 17 16   10 9 8 7 6 5 4 3 2 1

DEDICATION

To my parents, who taught me the value of learning; to my son, who motivated me to keep my goals in perspective; to my grandson, who brings me endless joy; and to all my nursing students, who inspired me to become the educator I am.

Maria C. Fressola, EdD, EdM, MA, RN, CNE
Professor of Nursing
Bergen Community College
Paramus, New Jersey

This book is dedicated to educators all over the world and to clinical practitioners who are aiming to become future educators of the next generation of nurses, by exposing themselves to the pedagogy of teaching.

The book is also dedicated to my husband, Joe; my children, Tonia Ann and Kevin; and my large family of sisters, brothers, and cousins who made this possible by their selfless support.

G. Elaine Patterson, EdD, EdM, MA, APN, CNE
Professor of Nursing
Ramapo College of New Jersey
Mahwah, New Jersey

Contents

Preface

The nursing shortage in the United States is well documented. Several reports by the American Association of Colleges of Nursing (AACN) reiterate that in recent years U.S. nursing schools have turned away thousands of qualified applicants from baccalaureate and graduate nursing programs due to an insufficient number of faculty, clinical sites, classroom space, clinical preceptors, and budget constraints. Nursing programs are challenged to devise creative and innovative means to bolster the nurse educator pool and decrease the national nursing shortage. One potential group of faculty can be found in the clinical practitioner pool, some of whom are awaiting the opportunity to transition into academic education.

This shortage of nursing educators has forced colleges and universities to hire master's-prepared nurses and nurse practitioners, who often have strong clinical backgrounds but are lacking in academic preparation and experience in teaching. To ensure that faculty are socialized into the profession and have the skills and know-how to teach, meet required competencies, and become effective teachers, colleges and universities are challenged to create environments wherein neophyte and inexperienced faculty can flourish. Neophyte faculty are expressing frustration with not really understanding the in-depth roles and responsibilities of faculty and not knowing where to go for guidance and other resources.

Additionally, clinical faculty who have been in the field—in some cases for decades—express the desire to move into academe but need the resources and guidance to be able to face the challenges in this unfamiliar area.

This book is intended as a response to the needs of neophytes as well as of experienced faculty who are looking for current information and strategies to include in their teaching repertoire.

Section I addresses the organizational world of academia. The section begins with discussions on how to view universities as organizations, with an emphasis on systems theory. Several types of academic institutions are described, and a variety of governance structures are outlined. Faculty roles and responsibilities are discussed, followed by ethical issues that one may confront during the course of teaching. The section ends by discussing the basic laws affecting student rights, followed by accreditation matters and an introduction to some of the professional nursing accreditation organizations.

Section II discusses classroom teaching. The emphasis on curriculum development is intentional because this is an area where clinicians often have the least experience. The process of developing a curriculum from the inception is intended to lay out for the educator the steps taken from beginning to end, from devising a mission statement to choosing a curriculum design, choosing an organizing framework, determining program outcomes and student learning outcomes, developing objectives, and devising evaluation strategies.

Internal and external factors influencing curriculum development are also discussed. The section summarizes a variety of teaching methods, differentiating between passive and active learning strategies. There is an exhaustive list of strategies from which the educator can draw, with examples of how to implement these strategies. The actual classroom environment plays a pivotal role in student learning. The reader is provided with information on how to manage the classroom, deal with the student and faculty codes of ethics, and develop learning communities. The section ends by discussing formative and summative evaluation strategies, developing test blueprints, developing test items, administering tests, and performing item analyses. There is also a discussion of faculty and student evaluation of program effectiveness.

Section III addresses clinical teaching. This section contains detailed information on how to select clinical sites, with a focus on different types of clinical agencies and how students are able to meet their objectives. Faculty responsibilities in choosing, preparing, and accompanying students to clinical sites are outlined. There also are discussions of ethical and legal issues in clinical teaching, along with HIPAA regulations and students' and patients' rights. A very detailed step-by-step approach to the process of clinical teaching provides the reader with quick access to planning and executing a typical clinical day. Finally, the section ends with some practical tips on evaluating the clinical experience formatively as well as summatively using concept maps, nursing care plans, evidence-based papers, journaling, observation, and feedback. Sample checklists are provided as well as hints on documenting student clinical performance.

The final section focuses on using technology in classrooms and clinical education. There is information on simulation, online pedagogy, and the integration of social media into traditional teaching. There also is an exhaustive list of technology resources from which the educator can draw.

Reviewers

Julia Aucoin, DNS, RN-BC, CNE
Adjunct Faculty
Nova Southeastern University College
of Nursing
Durham, NC

Sharon Beasley, PhD, RN, CME
Advanced Facilitator
University of Phoenix
Salem, IL

Diane Campbell, RN, DNP-PHN, FNP-BC
Associate Professor
Tennessee State University
Nashville, TN

**Ruth A. Chaplen, RN, DNP, ACNS-BC,
AOCN**
Assistant Professor, Clinical
Wayne State University
Detroit, MI

Debbie Ciesielka, EdD, ANP-BC
Associate Professor and MSN Program
Coordinator
Clarion University of Pennsylvania
Pittsburgh, PA

**Deborah J. Clark, PhD, MBA, MSN,
RN, CNE**
BSN Program Director
ECPI University
Virginia Beach, VA

Doris Clark, PhD, RN, CNE
Assistant Professor
Bowie State University
Bowie, MD

Cynthia L. Cummings, EdD, MSN
Associate Professor, Program Director
for the Accelerated Nursing Program
University of North Florida
Jacksonville, FL

**Kim Curry-Lourenco, PhD, MSN,
MEd, RN**
Associate Professor
Coordinator of Instruction and
Technology
Tidewater Community College,
Beazley School of Nursing
Virginia Beach, VA

Linda J. Curtin, RN, PhD, CCRN
Faculty
University of Massachusetts–Boston
Boston, MA

Vera Dauffenbach, EdD, MSN, RN
Associate Professor
Bellin College
Green Bay, WI

Lisa A. Davis, PhD, RN, NC-BC
Associate Department Head—Grad
    Studies
West Texas A&M University
Canyon, TX

Stephanie S. DeBoor, PhD, RN, CCRN
Associate Director of Graduate Programs
    and Assistant Professor
University of Nevada, Reno, Orvis
    School of Nursing
Reno, NV

Diane D. DePew, PhD, RN-BC
Assistant Clinical Professor
Drexel University, College of Nursing
    and Health Professions
Edgewater, MD

Jill B. Derstine, EdD, RN, FAAN
Clinical Associate Professor
Drexel University
Philadelphia, PA

Kimberly DeSantis, PhD, RN
Assistant Professor of Nursing
Indiana University East
Williamsburg, IN

**Pamela B. Edwards, EdD, MSN, RN-BC,
    CNE, CENP**
Associate Chief Nursing Officer,
    Education
Duke University Health System
Durham, NC

Cindy Farris, PhD, MSN, MPH, RN, CNE
Assistant Professor; Associate Dean of
    Undergraduate Nursing Program
Indiana University East
Richmond, IN

**Elizabeth A. Gazza, PhD, RN, LCCE,
    FACCE**
Associate Professor of Nursing
University of North Carolina
    Wilmington
Wilmington, NC

**Elizabeth I. Hartman, PhD, MSN,
    RNC-OB, CNE**
Assistant Professor
West Coast University
North Hollywood, CA

Layna Himmelberg, RN, CNE
Associate Professor
Clarkson College
Omaha, NE

Jane Leach, PhD, RNC, CNE
Graduate Coordinator, MSN Programs
Midwestern State University
Wichita Falls, TX

Joanne McDermott, PhD, RN
Associate Professor
MidAmerican Nazarene University
Olathe, KS

Gerald Newberry, PhD
Assistant Professor of Nursing
Eastern Michigan University
Ypsilanti, MI

**George Peraza-Smith, DNP, GNP-BC,
  AGPCNP-C, CNE**
Associate Dean and Associate Professor
United States University, College of
  Nursing
Chula Vista, CA

Janna C. Roop, PhD, RN, CHPN
Assistant Professor (Clinical)
Wayne State University College
  of Nursing
Detroit, MI

Cathryn Tiller, RN, EdD
Faculty
Jacksonville University
Belle, MO

Bonnie White, MSN, RN, CNE, CCM
Assistant Professor
MCPHS University
Worcester, MA

**Edward "Buddy" Wiltcher, EdD,
  MSN, RN**
Assistant Professor of Nursing, Interim
  Coordinator for LPN-RN Mobility
  Program
Tennessee State University
Hendersonville, TN

Colleges and Universities

CHAPTER 1

The Organizational World of Academia

OBJECTIVES

- Examine the structure in your higher education institution and how it affects the governance process among administrators, staff, and faculty.
- Compare the mission and goals of various higher education colleges and universities and how they define the institutions' responsibilities for meeting the teaching, research, and scholarship needs for the communities they serve.
- Analyze the bylaws in your institution and their impact on academic operations related to faculty, students, and administrators.
- Examine your rights as a faculty member to academic freedom and collective bargaining.
- Design your plan for achieving rank, tenure, and promotion at your higher education institution by addressing your responsibilities in teaching, research, scholarship, and community service.
- Formulate your plan for achieving the NLN competencies for nurse educators.

THE TRANSITION FROM CLINICIAN TO FACULTY

You have been working as a healthcare provider for many years and now have decided to expand your professional goals by becoming an educator in the world of academia. You are ready to make the transition from a clinician in a healthcare setting to an educator in a college or university. Making this transition does not mean you have decided to give up your role as a healthcare provider. Instead, you are now ready to help others learn how to become knowledgeable and safe practitioners who possess the clinical judgment and reasoning necessary to promote and maintain the health and wellness of society.

The education of nursing students in the nursing program requires faculty to create a balance between theoretical knowledge and clinical application. This vital role is a formidable challenge that requires you, a clinical expert, to now expand your abilities by adapting your instructional methodologies to address different student learning styles. This is not an easy task.

By taking on this new role as faculty, you also become a learner. You are now part of a different environment unfamiliar to you. The players in this environment are mostly faculty just like you. This organizational world of academia is different from the healthcare environment you have come to know throughout your years of employment. As a new faculty member within the college community, it is important for you to know and understand the dynamics of this environment and how you can learn to fit and develop within this structure.

This book will help you with this transition. You will be presented with a view of colleges and universities as organizations whose missions and goals focus on the educational needs of various student groups. You will be able to explore the governance of academic institutions, review legal considerations in higher education, address all aspects of curriculum and teaching, understand how institutions utilize committee structure to govern, and learn how to succeed in this ever-changing, dynamic environment.

COLLEGES AND UNIVERSITIES AS ORGANIZATIONS

As a nurse, you are familiar with many nursing professional associations. Now that you have decided to enter the world of academia, you should familiarize yourself with the American Association of University Professors (AAUP) because this organization is the voice for faculty members in higher education. Founded in 1915 by Arthur Lovejoy and John Dewey, the AAUP remains the leading organization dedicated to the development of standards and procedures that maintain quality in higher education and the protection of academic freedom in colleges and universities. The mission of the AAUP is as follows:

> . . . to advance academic freedom and shared governance; to define fundamental professional values and standards for higher education, to promote the economic security of faculty, the academic professionals, graduate students, post-doctoral fellows, and all those engaged in teaching and research in higher education; to help the higher education community to organize to make our goals a reality; and to ensure higher education's contribution to the common good. . . . (American Association of University Professors, n.d.)

In 2013, the AAUP reorganized into three interlocking divisions under the AAUP umbrella: the American Association of University Professors (AAUP), the American Association of University Professors Collective Bargaining Congress (AAUP-CBC), and the AAUP Foundation. The AAUP is a nonprofit professional organization formed to define professional values and standards for higher education while protecting academic freedom and promoting shared governance in colleges and universities. The AAUP-CBC is the organizing and collective bargaining unit for tenured faculty, tenure-track faculty, and academic professionals that defends fairer procedures for resolving grievances and secures the academic and economic security of faculty and professionals in the academic community. The AAUP Foundation is a nonprofit charitable organization created to promote the educational functions of the AAUP.

The educational policies created by the AAUP are committed to academic freedom and shared governance and set the direction for the professional values and standards adopted in higher education. You will learn more about the influence AAUP has had on the structure and operations of higher education as you proceed through this chapter.

Organizational Systems

All organizations are social units structured to manage the needs of the system while pursuing collective goals. Members of these organizations have assigned roles, responsibilities, and authority to carry out different tasks. Colleges and universities also are social units, but differ in many ways from other organizations in their management, leadership, and governance.

Colleges and universities are open systems made up of two subsystems, technical and administrative. Each of these subsystems has inputs and outputs that interact with each other to achieve the mission of the institution. The technical subsystem is composed of inputs such as students, faculty, academic freedom policies, and programs that produce outputs such as graduates, service, and prestige. The administrative subsystem includes regulations, budgets, and administrative personnel that direct the organization. These two subsystems interact with each other, and a change in one subsystem may change the direction of the college or university. These subsystems are responsive to each other, but each maintains its own identity. These subsystems within institutions of higher education are also responsive to the economic, social, and political needs of the environment with which they must interact.

To understand how these subsystems interact with each other, we need to consider how they are connected and the extent to which these subsystems share internal processes and structures. These connections may be loosely or tightly coupled interactions that are likely to occur between these subsystems in their attempts to meet the needs of the environment. In a tightly coupled system we can observe situations in which a change in one situation directly causes changes in the other system. In contrast, systems that are loosely coupled are still responsive to each other but may preserve their own identities and separateness. In a loosely coupled system, coordination of activities is problematic and makes administrative change more difficult. In the open system of colleges or universities, "everything cannot be tightly coupled to everything else, and loose coupling between and within subsystems is more prevalent than tight coupling" (Birnbaum, 1991, p. 41). This loose coupling between the administrative and technical subsystems makes innovation possible through the autonomous actions of many individuals and the general lack of management controls. Loose coupling is an adaptive device needed for the survival of an open system, and a structure administration may need to understand and accept it for the advancement of the organization (Weick, 1976).

It is beyond the scope of this book to explore the advantages and disadvantages of tightly and loosely coupled educational systems. What is important is for you to understand the dynamic structure of the institution resulting from the relationships between the technical and administrative subsystems. You also need to consider the roles and decision-making responsibilities of these two subsystems and how the economic, social, and political forces within the environment may influence the responsibilities of both subsystems.

Mission and Goals

Colleges and universities are involved with meeting the teaching, research, scholarship, and service responsibilities they were created to achieve (Hudson, 2013). These responsibilities are very different from those in the corporate world. Teaching involves the development of academic programs containing curriculum to prepare individuals for lifetime careers, classroom instruction, assessment of learning, counseling, and advisement. Research in the academic world is aimed at making new discoveries with the help of external funding through grants and financial incentives. Service to the community by academic institutions may include consulting services to community agencies to help address community needs, providing continuing education workshops to professionals, and creating service learning projects that integrate community service with instruction while fostering civic responsibility and strengthening communities.

These responsibilities are perceived differently depending on the population the academic institution was created to serve. Some institutions may give more attention to teaching and service learning, whereas others emphasize research and scholarship. An institution's purpose is usually stated in its mission statement and goals. As a new faculty member, it is important for you to review the institution's mission and goals to determine where the institution places the most emphasis. This will alert you to the expectations you will encounter in your role as a faculty member in this institution of higher education.

The nursing program also has a mission statement and/or philosophy that should be congruent with the mission and goals of the institution. This mission statement guides curriculum development and planning of educational activities. The mission and goals of a nursing program will differ depending on the level of nursing education and the type of degree awarded. In addition to a mission statement, some nursing programs may have a philosophy containing the common elements of the nursing metaparadigm: nurse, patient, environment, and health (Billings & Halstead, 2016). A nursing program's mission statement and philosophy are developed by the faculty and reviewed periodically as changes occur within the nursing profession subsequent to changes in scope of practice within the profession.

Types of Academic Institutions

There are three basic types of academic institutions you need to be familiar with: community colleges, four-year liberal arts colleges, and universities. The type of institution will determine its mission, goals, and student learning outcomes. As faculty, you need to have an understanding of the different types of institutions, their history, their size, and their sources of financial assistance. A comprehensive source for this information is the Carnegie Foundation for the Advancement of Teaching (www.carnegiefoundation.org).

Community colleges, sometimes referred to as junior colleges or technical colleges, are two-year institutions with a mission of providing higher education and lower-level tertiary education by awarding certificates or associate degrees. Community colleges may also offer noncredit continuing education and adult education courses, remedial education for high school graduates who are not academically ready to enroll in college-level courses, and industrial training contracted with local companies that pay the college to provide specific training for their employees. After graduating from a community college, students with an associate degree may directly enter the workforce or transfer to a four-year liberal arts college or university to complete a bachelor's degree. Schools often have transfer and/or articulation agreements explaining the transfer credit agreement and teaching location for upper division courses. In some transfer/articulation agreements, students may obtain a bachelor's degree without leaving the community college campus.

The main purpose of community colleges is to provide academic, vocational, and professional education. In the technical subsystems, most faculty who teach in community colleges have a minimum of a master's degree with expertise in a specialty area, whereas employees within the administrative subsystem often have a doctorate degree with previous teaching experience in higher education.

Most community college systems are publicly run institutions of higher learning supported by local and state funding. Student enrollment impacts the amount of funding the community college will receive to operate its fiscal budget. Attempts are made to curtail tuition costs per student, but the strength of these attempts will depend on the amount of state funding the community college receives.

Traditional four-year colleges and universities offer students the opportunity to obtain a bachelor of arts or bachelor of science degree in their chosen field of study.

Universities may also be structured to include a liberal arts college as well as other specialized colleges or graduate schools that enable students to obtain a master's degree. Private four-year colleges and universities are generally smaller than public institutions and rely on tuition, fees, and private sources of funding. Public institutions receive funding from local and state governments; therefore, tuition costs for students living in-state will be lower than tuition costs for out-of-state residents. Faculty employed in the technical subsystems of four-year colleges and universities have earned doctorate degrees in their area of specialty. Research is encouraged in these higher education institutions as a means for acquiring increased funding for the college or university.

ACADEMIC ADMINISTRATION AND GOVERNANCE

The administrative structure of most colleges and universities is made up of a board of trustees; a president or chancellor; an academic vice president, often referred to as a provost; and several vice presidents for different departments. The board of trustees is charged with the ultimate responsibility for the overall operations of the institution— the fiduciary responsibility, the continuation of the institution's mission and goals, setting institutional policies, and serving as the legal agents of their institution in litigation cases involving higher education and the law. Boards are also charged with overseeing the selection and hiring of the college or university president in addition to making final decisions with regard to hiring, reappointment, tenure, promotion, and sabbaticals.

The president or chancellor is the administrative head of the organization and reports directly to the board of trustees. The president is the executive leadership of the organization; he or she advises the board on policies and other matters necessary to run the institution smoothly. The president ensures sound fiscal management and represents the college to the community, the state, and federal agencies.

In many schools, the academic vice president (VP) often serves as the provost; he or she answers directly to the president and is responsible for the administrative support and functionality of the organization. This role often involves ensuring that the organization stays true to its mission. The VP or provost also is responsible for curricular oversight, instructional integrity, and research efforts. Often deans and other vice presidents answer to the academic VP and/or the provost. Your school may have several vice presidents, depending on the size of the institution (e.g., vice president of administration services, vice president of institutional effectiveness, vice president of student affairs, vice president of human resources), and deans of the schools or divisions. It is important for you to be familiar with the administrative structure and where the nursing program fits within this structure.

Most colleges and universities may be further organized into schools or divisions containing different academic departments. For example, the nursing program may be a school or college within the university or it may be a department within the school of health professions. There are many variations in the organizational structures of colleges and universities, and it is important for you to understand these structures and the reporting mechanisms for the nursing program.

The concept of governance reflects a major difference between how institutions of higher education and other organizations function to achieve their missions and goals. Although there is no one accepted definition for governance, the term has been addressed by the AAUP in terms of structure, legal relationships, authority patterns, rights and responsibilities, and decision-making processes. A *governance system* refers to the structures and processes through which institutional members interact with and influence each other while communicating within the larger environment (Birnbaum, 1991). The 1966 Statement on Government of Colleges and Universities issued jointly by the American Association of University Professors, the American Council on Education, and the Association of Governing Boards of Universities and Colleges addresses some of the principles of governance as a shared responsibility among governing board members, faculty, and students (AAUP, 1966).

Shared governance is a delicate balance between faculty and staff participation in planning and decision making on the one hand and administrative accountability on the other hand. Although shared governance attempts to give various groups of elected people a voice in key decision-making processes, it may not necessarily give these groups the ultimate authority for the final decision. The ultimate responsibility for decision making on issues involving the academic institution rests with the president and/or the governing board.

Within colleges and universities there is a faculty senate that is the governing body for academic issues. The senate participates in decision making on all academic and student affairs matters related to the operation of the college or university (Hubbell, 2010). The faculty senate formulates resolutions and recommendations and advises the president of the college or university on matters of importance to the governance and operation of the institution. Within the faculty senate there may be several subcommittees to help the senate carry out its functions and operations. Examples of these subcommittees may include Academic Standing, Admissions, and Curriculum.

There are differences in the level of faculty governance among colleges and universities, so you should take the time to review the governance structure where you are presently employed. This may help you come to a better understanding about how the board of trustees and administrators or the faculty maintain decision-making authority for the operations of the college or university. This information may be contained in the bylaws documents of the overall institution as well as the faculty bylaws.

Bylaws in Higher Education

Bylaws address the academic governance in institutions of higher education by providing definitions and guidelines addressing institutional operations related to faculty, students, administrators, and committee structures. Bylaws are the rules and regulations enacted by an institution of higher education to provide a framework for its operation and management. Bylaws are very specific for each institution and are intended to promote an understanding of the roles and responsibilities with respect to the university or college governing boards, committee structure, and faculty.

Bylaws define the rights the members have within the organization; how much power these members have to make decisions; and the rights, decision-making authority, and powers of the board. Bylaws provide an effective system for faculty and students to participate in the development of policies on academic matters. The rules contained within an institution's bylaws are so important that they may not be changed without a formal vote and an agreement by a majority of the members. Generally bylaws address the following:

- Composition of the faculty, their voting rights, and their role in academic governance
- Composition of the student body and their participation in academic governance
- Composition of the academic administrators, their appointment and evaluation process, and their role in academic governance
- Composition of the college or university academic governance committees, their functions, and their membership including student representatives and voting rights
- Composition of college- or university-level standing committees; their function, policies, and procedures; membership; and lines of accountability to other academic governance committees
- Establishment of ad hoc committees, the method of selecting members, and their functions and procedures
- Composition of student–faculty judiciaries and the academic appeals board, and their policies, procedures, and membership

Institutional bylaws may also contain specific faculty policies addressing, but not limited to, the following: academic freedom; tenure and promotion; faculty responsibilities; compensation including benefits, leaves of absence, sabbaticals, and retirement; legal matters; and grievance procedures. The bylaws may also include specific college and university policies addressing the rights and conduct of all employees (O'Neil, 2014).

Each academic unit within a college or university also has bylaws that are consistent with the policies established by the board of trustees and conform to the policies and procedures contained within the institutional bylaws. Together, institutional bylaws and the bylaws of the academic unit provide an effective system for promoting an understanding of the roles and responsibilities of the college community with respect to the mission of education, research/scholarship, and service.

Nursing bylaws conform to institutional bylaws and provide a democratic organization of the governance structure for the faculty in the nursing department or school of nursing. The faculty is organized as a policy-setting body that participates in decision making regarding the implementation of policies related to the educational, research, and practice/management activities within the nursing program. Through their membership on nursing committees, faculty perform those academic functions essential to the operations of the nursing program and student welfare. Generally nursing bylaws will address faculty organizational structure, duties and voting rights, and the composition and function of various faculty committees. Faculty standing committees may include, but are not limited to, the following:

- Faculty assembly
- Faculty executive council
- Admissions and academic standards for baccalaureate and graduate programs
- Appointment, promotion, and tenure
- Curriculum
- Academic standards
- Assessment and evaluation
- Faculty practice and community engagement
- Student matters
- Scholarships/awards and recruitment
- Special subcommittees/ad hoc committees
- Research and scholarship

It is very important for you to become knowledgeable about the bylaws of the college or university as well as the nursing school or department. These two documents will be your guide to being an effective and successful member of the college community.

Participation on College Committees

Faculty in colleges and universities are expected to become active members in the college community by contributing their expertise to various college activities that promote the mission and goals of the institution. Faculty responsibilities expand beyond the classroom to membership on various college committees. These college-wide committees are developed to address the needs of students during their college experience. Membership on these committees is usually made up of faculty from various disciplines throughout the college who volunteer to serve as committee members for a specific period of time. In some cases, membership on these college-wide committees is an elected position. These committees meet on a regular basis to address issues currently affecting the students and the college. In addition to college-wide committees, there are department committees. These committees are designed to address student needs and professional issues affecting the specific discipline. As faculty, you may be elected by your colleagues in nursing to be a committee chairperson or you may volunteer for this important responsibility.

Academic Freedom

One term you are sure to hear early in your new career is *academic freedom*. Experienced faculty will always refer to this term to defend their academic activities. So what does it mean?

Academic freedom is a basic right of faculty in higher education. This intellectual freedom is derived from the nature of the quest for knowledge and extends to institutions of higher education. Institutions of higher education are conducted for the common good, not to further the special interests of individual faculty or the institution. The 1940 Statement of Principles on Academic Freedom and Tenure states that academic freedom applies to both teaching and research (AAUP, 1940). Academic freedom protects the rights of the teacher in teaching and the rights of the student in learning. The principles of academic freedom include the following:

- Faculty are entitled to full freedom in research and in the publication of the results.
- Faculty are entitled to freedom in the classroom when discussing their subject but should be careful not to introduce controversial material that has no relationship to their subject.
- Faculty are citizens, members of a learned profession, and officers of an educational institution. When they speak or write as citizens, they are free from institutional censorship or discipline and should not represent themselves as spokespersons for the institution.

Academic freedom also includes the rights of faculty to retain the rights to their intellectual property; to participate in the governance of the college or university; to advance in their profession without fear of discrimination; and to criticize administrators, trustees, and other public officials without recrimination (Association of American Colleges and Universities, 2006).

Within the nursing profession, the board of nursing's (BON's) rules and regulations for nursing programs address nursing faculty responsibilities for program curriculum. Nursing faculty qualifications to teach within a nursing program are well documented by the BON and include the responsibility to develop, implement, teach, and evaluate the curriculum. Through their use of academic freedom, nursing faculty are able to choose a philosophy and organizing framework, decide program objectives and outcomes, and design the entire nursing program curriculum.

Unionization and Collective Bargaining in Higher Education

The presence of faculty governance in colleges and universities does not preclude the need for or the usefulness of collective bargaining through unionization. Collective bargaining through unionization is designed to protect academic freedom, to establish and strengthen faculty governance in institutions of higher education, and to provide fair procedures for resolving faculty grievances.

Public colleges and universities have unions to negotiate the collective bargaining rights of faculty and staff; private colleges are not compelled to allow faculty unionization (American Association of University Professors, n.d.). Members of the collective bargaining units within the college or university are subject to compulsory annual dues and are given the right to elect union leadership. When faculties choose collective bargaining, the board of trustees and administration have a collaborative obligation to bargain in good faith with the faculty-elected union representatives to achieve mutual agreement on employee issues.

If you are employed in a public college or university that has a union representing faculty, you need to become familiar with the union contract. This contract usually contains faculty contractual agreements for teaching load; criteria for promotion, reappointment, tenure, fringe benefits, and salary scales; and grievance procedures. If you are a faculty member in a nonunion environment, you may find this information in other official college or university documents such as the faculty handbook or bylaws. It is also a good idea to review similar documents prepared for faculty by the AAUP—for example, the Statement on Collective Bargaining formulated by the AAUP (2009).

Faculty Tenure, Rank, and Promotion

At the time of your employment as faculty, you may be placed on a probationary status requiring annual reappointment until you have achieved tenure. The probationary period is usually defined by the institution, but is not to exceed seven years. Tenure is a continuing, indefinite, or permanent appointment granted to a faculty member subsequent to a probationary period and extensive objective peer and administrative review. This concept of tenure has been extensively debated in the higher education literature. A more extensive review of the literature on the topic of tenure in higher education can be found at www.aaup.org (click on Reports & Publications, and then AAUP Policies & Reports).

Sometimes, at the time of your appointment the college or university may offer you the choice of pursuing a tenured or nontenured position. If you have been hired for a tenure-track position, the college or university is willing to commit to your continued employment until retirement, provided you have satisfied your faculty obligations during the probationary period. During your probationary period you need to devote time to professional activities aimed at academic scholarship while becoming involved in college affairs affecting the college community. For example, you may volunteer for participation in college-wide committees; student activities, such as being an advisor to a student club; or participation in faculty development programs, or you may apply for grant money for research or program development purposes and writing for publication. The rigor with which you may need to pursue these scholarly activities depends on the mission and goals of the institution and may vary among the community college setting and the four-year college or university environment.

Regardless of whether you chose a tenure-track or non–tenure-track position, you need to completely understand the academic requirements for each of these appointments as well as your intended professional goals. If you have chosen a tenure-track position, it is likely you will have anywhere between five and seven years to achieve this tenure. Unfortunately, if you choose this track and are not successful in receiving tenure, the college or university can end your employment at the institution.

In most cases, tenure cannot be transferred from one institution to another. However, if you are teaching at one institution for several years in a tenure-track position and then leave that institution before being granted tenure, those years of teaching may count toward your tenure years at your new place of employment. The college or university administration decides if your previous years of teaching in a tenure-track faculty position at another institution will count toward your tenure years at the new institution. Your achievements with previous research, publications, and grants also are strong factors in deciding if your previous years in academia will count toward your present tenure status.

Remember, your faculty appointment is a probationary one subject to annual administrative approval by the board of trustees until you receive tenure. As hard as you may try for tenure through your scholarly endeavors during your probationary period, receiving tenure at an institution is not guaranteed. If you do not receive tenure after your probationary period, the college or university may give you a terminal contract lasting one year.

At times, even tenured faculty may be terminated for adequate cause or extraordinary circumstances of financial exigencies. For this reason, dismissal and grievance procedures exist in institutions of higher education to ensure academic due process. Colleges and universities have policies and agreements in place related to faculty and institutional working relationships. Most of the policies and agreements formulated by colleges and universities emanate from the Association of American Colleges' and the American Association of University Professors' written key policy statements on tenure and termination of employment. The AAUP has issued extensive ongoing position statements on faculty dismissal and grievance procedures to support academic due process for faculty (AAUP, 1958).

Some colleges and universities may hire faculty for only non–tenure-track positions. These faculty may be appointed because of their skills and expertise in nonacademic careers and usually receive renewal contracts for periods of time determined by the institution. If the administration decides not to renew a nontenured faculty contract, the faulty member involved is informed of the decision in writing by the individual making the decision and may request a formal review of the reasons for the decision. Reasons for termination of appointments by the institution may include, but are not limited to, discontinuance of a program or department of instruction and financial exigency (AAUP, 2013).

Faculty are also eligible for promotion to higher ranks within the college or university. The qualifications for these ranks are clearly defined and include the educational degree and experience needed for the position. These ranks, in ascending order, include instructor, assistant professor, associate professor, and full professor. Some colleges appoint faculty to a lecturer position, but these individuals may not have the same rights and privileges as those faculty appointed to rank. Some departments, including nursing, may hire adjunct, clinical, or part-time faculty on a semester-to-semester basis for specific teaching assignments. These positions usually do not have the benefits of a faculty ranked position.

As a new faculty member, you need to become familiar with the academic requirements for reappointment during your probationary status and promotion from one rank to the next. You need to carefully review these official documents because the requirements differ among colleges and universities. For example, in a union environment, the union contract may identify the degree requirements, number of years with college-level experience, and number of years in present rank before you may apply for promotion to another rank. Similar procedures may be followed in private colleges and universities.

Once you have satisfied the criteria for promotion to a higher rank, your application for promotion is given to the promotion committee. This committee reviews your application for adherence to the criteria for the rank you have applied for as well as your academic accomplishments in the previous rank. Usually colleges and universities are allocated a certain number of promotions annually to each rank depending on the institution's budget. Your attempt to achieve promotion to a higher rank is a competitive process. Members of the promotion committee diligently review all applications for promotion together with the applicants' academic achievements. Depending on the procedure for granting promotion, these applicants may be placed in rank order, and those with the highest rank are considered for promotion. If those with the highest rank outnumber the allocated promotion positions for that specific rank, then the committee members usually vote on the final decision. If you are denied promotion in one year, you are free to reapply the following year. The recommended promotions decided upon by the promotion committee are sent to the board of trustees for their final approval.

FACULTY RESPONSIBILITIES IN THE WORLD OF ACADEMIA

Faculty responsibilities in the world of academia fall into four broad categories: teaching, research, scholarship, and community service. If you are working in a union environment, these responsibilities are explained in the union contract. You need to be very familiar with the union contract for your institution because contracts may vary among two-year community colleges and four-year colleges and universities. Non-union institutions of higher education also have official documents such as faculty bylaws and a faculty handbook that outline faculty responsibilities. It is also a good idea to review some of the documents prepared by the AAUP to learn more about the rights and responsibilities of faculty in higher education.

Teaching and Student Services

The basic academic teaching year is assigned over 32 weeks, usually beginning September 1 and ending June 30. For this reason, full-time faculty are considered 10-month employees. This academic year is usually composed of two 16-week semesters, Fall and Spring, although some colleges and universities have adopted semesters of different lengths as well as summer and winter intercessions.

As a 10-month employee, teaching credit hours during these 32 weeks are considered in-load hours and may vary from 24 to 30 teaching credit hours per academic year. Teaching credit hours are determined by the student credit hours defined by a given course; for example, if a course is worth three credits toward a student's degree requirements, this course will meet for approximately three hours weekly. Faculty will teach this course for three hours weekly throughout the semester and receive three teaching hours toward their faculty load requirements. Therefore, teaching credit hours equal student credit hours. Also, teaching credit load usually requires faculty to set aside blocks of time for office hours for student appointments. If faculty teach more than the required 24 to 30 teaching credit hours, this is considered overload hours, and faculty are paid additional monies for this overload. Teaching during the summer and winter intercessions may also be considered overload hours.

In summary, faculty workload may be met through various load and overload teaching credit hours. As a 10-month employee, your salary is determined by your rank in the institution as well as the number of required teaching load credit hours. When faculty engage in teaching responsibilities beyond the required teaching credit hours, this time is considered overload, and faculty are compensated on a prorated basis. When faculty engage in nonteaching responsibilities with managerial approval, these may be credited toward the required teaching credit hours. Alternatively, they may be credited above the required teaching credit hours, in which case faculty are compensated. It is very important for you to review your faculty contract regarding wages and compensation.

Mentoring and academic advisement of students are other nonteaching responsibilities expected from faculty. During this time faculty are expected to be available to help students with decisions regarding their professional goals. In some situations, if students are having difficulty with coursework, faculty are also expected to help with tutoring needs. Often these nonteaching responsibilities are scheduled during faculty office hours.

Research and Scholarship

Faculty may also be engaged in nonteaching scholarship activities that include preparing publications and research, special projects for the institution, or presentations at professional development conferences. These nonteaching activities may be credited toward the faculty's required credit hours, or faculty may be given the choice to receive these credit hours as overload. For example, in the mission statement and goals of some colleges and universities, research is an important and expected responsibility of faculty. In these institutions, teaching credit hours may be adjusted to allow faculty time for research activities that bring outside funding into the institution. Assignment of nonteaching activities credited toward faculty's required credit loads are usually subject to academic/managerial decisions by the college or university.

Community Service

Faculty can share their professional expertise both within and beyond the walls of the college or university by presenting at conferences. When faculty present at national conferences, they are representing the campus community to other constituencies. Active membership within professional organizations is another way faculty can represent the college or university on a national level.

Another way faculty can show support for their membership in the college community is by volunteering as a member of a taskforce designed to address special projects on campus. Faculty may apply for grant money from government and private agencies to help with the implementation of these special campus projects.

It is important for faculty to become active in the life of the campus community. It is not enough just to teach within your discipline and participate in discipline-specific activities. You need to reach out to other college constituencies and become involved in their activities. Your active involvement in the campus community may be the determining consideration in your promotion to a higher rank.

PREREQUISITES FOR BEING A NURSE EDUCATOR

A question most nurses ask is what the prerequisite is to becoming a nurse educator. You may be surprised to know that there is not a specific or unique list of criteria for someone wanting to become a nurse educator. So where should you begin? Educational requirements vary from program to program and state to state. It is generally understood that one should have a higher degree than the level being taught. For example, a bachelor of science in nursing (BSN)–prepared nurse may teach at the diploma nurse level, a master of science in nursing (MSN) nurse is able to teach at the BSN and diploma levels, and the doctor of philosophy (PhD) can teach at all levels of nursing. This, however, does not hold true at most schools because schools make decisions on who they want to teach their students based on established national guidelines and competencies. The National League for Nursing (NLN) has a list of competencies for the nurse educator that can be found at www.nln.org. The following eight competencies with interpretative statements can be used as a guide for the nurse educator and are often used as a means for evaluating the effectiveness of nurse educators.

Competency 1: Facilitate Learning

Nurse educators are responsible for creating an environment in classroom, laboratory, and clinical settings that facilitates student learning and the achievement of desired cognitive, affective, and psychomotor outcomes. To facilitate learning effectively, the nurse educator:

- Implements a variety of teaching strategies appropriate to learner needs, desired learner outcomes, content, and context
- Grounds teaching strategies in educational theory and evidence-based teaching practices
- Recognizes multicultural, gender, and experiential influences on teaching and learning
- Engages in self-reflection and continued learning to improve teaching practices that facilitate learning
- Uses information technologies skillfully to support the teaching/learning process

- Practices skilled oral, written, and electronic communication that reflects an awareness of self and others, along with an ability to convey ideas in a variety of contexts
- Models critical and reflective thinking
- Creates opportunities for learners to develop their critical thinking and critical reasoning skills
- Shows enthusiasm for teaching, learning, and nursing that inspires and motivates students
- Demonstrates interest in and respect for learners
- Uses personal attributes (e.g., caring, confidence, patience, integrity, and flexibility) that facilitate learning
- Develops collegial working relationships with students, faculty colleagues, and clinical agency personnel to promote positive learning environments
- Maintains the professional practice knowledge base needed to help learners prepare for contemporary nursing practice
- Serves as a role model of professional nursing

Competency 2: Facilitate Learner Development and Socialization

Nurse educators recognize their responsibility for helping students develop as nurses and integrate the values and behaviors expected of those who fulfill that role. To facilitate learner development and socialization effectively, the nurse educator:

- Identifies individual learning styles and unique learning needs of international, adult, multicultural, educationally disadvantaged, physically challenged, at-risk, and second-degree learners
- Provides resources to diverse learners that help meet their individual learning needs
- Engages in effective advisement and counseling strategies that help learners meet their professional goals
- Creates learning environments that are focused on socialization to the role of the nurse and facilitate learners' self-reflection and personal goal setting
- Fosters the cognitive, psychomotor, and affective development of learners
- Recognizes the influence of teaching styles and interpersonal interactions on learner outcomes
- Assists learners to develop the ability to engage in thoughtful and constructive self and peer evaluation
- Models professional behaviors for learners including, but not limited to, involvement in professional organizations, engagement in lifelong learning activities, dissemination of information through publications and presentations, and advocacy

Competency 3: Use Assessment and Evaluation Strategies

Nurse educators use a variety of strategies to assess and evaluate student learning in classroom, laboratory, and clinical settings, as well as in all domains of learning. To use assessment and evaluation strategies effectively, the nurse educator:

- Uses extant literature to develop evidence-based assessment and evaluation practices
- Uses a variety of strategies to assess and evaluate learning in the cognitive, psychomotor, and affective domains
- Implements evidence-based assessment and evaluation strategies that are appropriate to the learner and to learning goals
- Uses assessment and evaluation data to enhance the teaching/learning process
- Provides timely, constructive, and thoughtful feedback to learners
- Demonstrates skill in the design and use of tools for assessing clinical practice

Competency 4: Participate in Curriculum Design and Evaluation of Program Outcomes

Nurse educators are responsible for formulating program outcomes and designing curricula that reflect contemporary healthcare trends and prepare graduates to function effectively in the healthcare environment. They ensure that the curriculum reflects institutional philosophy and mission, current nursing and healthcare trends, and community and societal needs so as to prepare graduates for practice in a complex, dynamic, multicultural healthcare environment. To participate effectively in curriculum design and the evaluation of program outcomes, the nurse educator:

- Demonstrates knowledge of curriculum development including identifying program outcomes, developing competency statements, writing learning objectives, and selecting appropriate learning activities and evaluation strategies
- Bases curriculum design and implementation decisions on sound educational principles, theory, and research
- Revises the curriculum based on assessment of program outcomes, learner needs, and societal and healthcare trends
- Implements curricular revisions using appropriate change theories and strategies
- Creates and maintains community and clinical partnerships that support educational goals
- Collaborates with external constituencies throughout the process of curriculum revision
- Designs and implements program assessment models that promote continuous quality improvement of all aspects of the program

Competency 5: Function as a Change Agent and Leader

Nurse educators function as change agents and leaders to create a preferred future for nursing education and nursing practice. To function effectively as a change agent and leader, the nurse educator:

- Models cultural sensitivity when advocating for change
- Integrates a long-term, innovative, and creative perspective into the nurse educator role
- Participates in interdisciplinary efforts to address healthcare and educational needs locally, regionally, nationally, or internationally
- Evaluates organizational effectiveness in nursing education
- Implements strategies for organizational change
- Provides leadership in the parent institution as well as in the nursing program to enhance the visibility of nursing and its contributions to the academic community
- Promotes innovative practices in educational environments
- Develops leadership skills to shape and implement change

Competency 6: Pursue Continuous Quality Improvement in the Nurse Educator Role

Nurse educators recognize that their role is multidimensional and that an ongoing commitment to develop and maintain competence in the role is essential. To pursue continuous quality improvement in the nurse educator role, the individual:

- Demonstrates a commitment to lifelong learning
- Recognizes that career enhancement needs and activities change as experience is gained in the role
- Participates in professional development opportunities that increase one's effectiveness in the role
- Balances the teaching, scholarship, and service demands inherent in the role of educator and member of an academic institution
- Uses feedback gained from self, peer, student, and administrative evaluation to improve role effectiveness
- Engages in activities that promote one's socialization to the role
- Uses knowledge of legal and ethical issues relevant to higher education and nursing education as a basis for influencing, designing, and implementing policies and procedures related to students, faculty, and the educational environment
- Mentors and supports faculty colleagues

Competency 7: Engage in Scholarship

Nurse educators acknowledge that scholarship is an integral component of the faculty role and that teaching itself is a scholarly activity. To engage effectively in scholarship, the nurse educator:

- Draws on extant literature to design evidence-based teaching and evaluation practices
- Exhibits a spirit of inquiry about teaching and learning, student development, evaluation methods, and other aspects of the role
- Designs and implements scholarly activities in an established area of expertise
- Disseminates nursing and teaching knowledge to a variety of audiences through various means
- Demonstrates skill in proposal writing for initiatives that include, but are not limited to, research, resource acquisition, program development, and policy development
- Demonstrates qualities of a scholar: integrity, courage, perseverance, vitality, and creativity

Competency 8: Function Within the Educational Environment

Nurse educators are knowledgeable about the educational environment within which they practice and recognize how political, institutional, social, and economic forces impact their role. To function as a good "citizen of the academy," the nurse educator:

- Uses knowledge of history and current trends and issues in higher education as a basis for making recommendations and decisions on educational issues
- Identifies how social, economic, political, and institutional forces influence higher education in general and nursing education in particular
- Develops networks, collaborations, and partnerships to enhance nursing's influence within the academic community
- Determines his or her own professional goals within the context of academic nursing and the mission of the parent institution and nursing program
- Integrates the values of respect, collegiality, professionalism, and caring to build an organizational climate that fosters the development of students and teachers
- Incorporates the goals of the nursing program and the mission of the parent institution when proposing change or managing issues
- Assumes a leadership role in various levels of institutional governance
- Advocates for nursing and nursing education in the political arena[1]

---

[1]Reproduced from National League for Nursing. (2005). *Core competencies of nurse educators with task statements.* National League for Nursing. All rights reserved.

These are not, however, the only competencies and expectations of the nurse educator. The American Association of Colleges of Nursing (AACN) also has competencies and expectations that are similar to those just listed. As detailed as these may seem, do not be overwhelmed. It is not expected that any one educator will immediately become competent in all these areas, but they are worth striving for during one's academic career. In addition to these established competencies, the AACN has developed competencies "designed to enhance the ability of nurse faculty to effectively develop quality and safety competencies among nurse graduates of their programs" (AACN, 2012). The 2012 AACN report is a summary of outcomes of programs held in 2010 and 2011 that gave nurse faculty the training and information necessary to improve their curricula. The report discussed six core competencies that were the focus of the training: patient-centered care, teamwork and collaboration, evidence-based practice, quality improvement, safety, and informatics. These topics will be expanded on throughout this text.

CERTIFIED NURSE EDUCATOR (CNE)

You may have noticed that some nurse educators have the initials *CNE* behind their names. In 2005, the National League for Nursing (NLN) instituted the Certified Nurse Educator credential, also known as the CNE. This credential recognizes nurse educators who are experienced and skilled in their role as nurse educator. The goal of the NLN was to recognize "excellence in the advanced specialty role of the academic nurse educator" (NLN, 2016). The prerequisites have changed over time; updated information can be found on the NLN website at www.nln.org. Basically, one must have at least two years of teaching experience in an academic setting, hold at least a master's-level degree, be licensed to practice within a state, and have successfully completed the certifying examination. The certification is good for five years, at which time the person is eligible to sit for recertification. As of 2014, there were more than 4500 CNEs. For some schools this is a requirement for teaching in their nursing programs. For others it is a mark of achievement, but not necessarily a requirement. In 2014, the NLN CNE program received five-year accreditation from the Institute of Credentialing Excellence.

There are several ways one can prepare for the CNE examination. The NLN website offers a number of free resources including a CNE Candidate handbook. Several CNE prep courses are offered by different nursing schools and taught by experts in the field. These are listed on the NLN website. You may also purchase one of the available CNE preparation texts. These texts follow the test blueprint of the core competencies and are supported by relevant research. The sample questions at the end of each chapter will no doubt be useful to anyone planning to take the examination.

MEMBERSHIP IN PROFESSIONAL ORGANIZATIONS

It is an expectation that educators will become members and support their professional organizations. There is an exhaustive list of professional nursing organizations. Two that are directly related to the role of the nurse educator are the National League for Nursing (NLN) and the American Association of Colleges of Nursing (AACN). Most nursing programs hold institutional membership in one or both organizations, so all full-time educators within the program are listed as members. Before attempting to purchase an individual membership, ask your dean whether your school is a "member school." The benefits of professional membership in the AACN and the NLN are combined here:

- Professional development through participation in seminars and conferences that are offered throughout the year; special discounted rates for members at conferences
- Free educational material and other resources
- Free subscriptions to professional journals
- Organizational support in seeking research funding
- Obtaining information to help keep current regarding changes in nursing education
- Exposure to the legislative process and lobbying for funding
- Opportunity to participate on committees
- National recognition for accomplishments

SUMMARY

This chapter presented an overview of the structure and bylaws in institutions of higher education and how these structures and bylaws affect the governance process among administrators, staff, and faculty. Also included were important topics related to faculty rights, such as academic freedom and collective bargaining. The process for faculty to achieve rank, tenure, and promotion were reviewed. Finally, the competencies needed to be a certified nurse educator were identified.

CASE STUDIES

1. You are scheduled to interview for a faculty position in the nursing department at a nearby university. Consider the following, and create a list of questions related to them:
   a. The mission of the university
   b. Your rank at hire
   c. Requirements for receiving tenure and promotion

    d. Faculty in-load teaching requirements

    e. Faculty compensation

    f. Your responsibilities as a member of the college community

    g. The structure of shared governance at the university

2. You have been thinking seriously about achieving certification as a nurse educator. The NLN has developed eight competencies for evaluating the effectiveness of nurse educators. Review each of these competencies, and develop a plan for how you will meet these competencies in your professional faculty practice.

3. Now that you have entered the arena of higher education, decide which organizations you may want to join as an active member. These organizations may come from higher education, nursing education, or your professional practice. Explain why you chose each organization.

REFERENCES

American Association of Colleges and Universities. (n.d.) Yeshiva ruling. Retrived from http://www.aaup.org/import-tags/yeshiva-ruling

American Association of Colleges of Nursing. (2012). Quality and safety education for nurses. Retrieved from http://www.aacn.nche.edu/qsen/home

American Association of University Professors (AAUP). (1940). Statement of principles on academic freedom and tenure. Retrieved from http://www.aaup.org/report/1940-statement-principles-academic-freedom-and-tenure

American Association of University Professors (AAUP). (1958). Statement on procedural standards in faculty dismissal proceedings. Retrieved from http://www.aaup.org/report/statement-procedural-standards-faculty-dismissal-proceedings

American Association of University Professors (AAUP). (1966). Statement on government of colleges and universities. Retrieved from http://www.aaup.org/report/statement-government-colleges-and-universities

American Association of University Professors (AAUP). (2009). Statement on collective bargaining. Retrieved from http://www.aaup.org/AAUP/pubsres/policydocs/contents/statementcolbargaining.htm

American Association of University Professors (AAUP). (2013). Recommended institutional regulations on academic freedom and tenure. Retrieved from http://www.aaup.org/report/recommended-institutional-regulations-academic-freedom-and-tenure

Association of American Colleges and Universities. (2006). Academic freedom and educational responsibility. Retrieved from http://www.aacu.org/about/statements/academic-freedom

Billings, D. M., & Halstead, J. A. (2016). Clinical performance evaluation. In W. Bonnel (Ed.), *Teaching in nursing: A guide for faculty* (5th ed., pp. 449–466). St. Louis, MO: Elsevier/Saunders.

Birnbaum, R. (1991). *How Colleges Work*. San Francisco, CA: Jossey-Bass.

Hubbell, L. (2010, Fall). Thankless but vital: The role of the faculty senate chair. *Thought and Action*, 147–152.

Hudson, E. (2013). Educating for community change: Higher education's proposed role in community transformation through the federal promise neighborhood policy. *Journal of Higher Education Outreach and Engagement, 17*(3), 109–138.

National League for Nursing. (2016). Homepage. Retrieved from http://nln.org

O'Neil, R. (2013). Updating board bylaws—and beyond. *Trusteeship, 21*(2), 17–21.

Weick, K. E. (1976). Educational organizations as loosely coupled systems. *Administrative Science Quarterly, 21*, 1–19.

CHAPTER 2

Legal Issues and Accreditation in Higher Education

OBJECTIVES

- Apply the basic laws affecting student rights to your responsibilities as faculty.
- Analyze the impact of F-1 visas on students' progression in the nursing program.
- Explain students' right to challenge their grades.
- Identify nursing program admission requirements related to admission testing, criminal background checks, health clearance, liability insurance, certifications, and general education courses.
- Explain the accreditation process in higher education and the roles of the national agencies involved in this process.
- Interpret the NCLEX-RN test plan and its application to your role as a faculty member in an undergraduate nursing program.

The law in higher education is a highly specialized area containing extensive documents addressing student, faculty, college, and university rights and obligations in society. As a faculty member, you will be faced with a vast array of legal issues that arise in nursing education. Faculty often struggle with ways to solve some of the legal issues they confront in the classroom and the clinical setting. Navigating the legal issues every faculty member may face at some point in their professional career is a daunting task that requires, at a minimum, some understanding of the basic laws in higher education that can impact your role as faculty. This chapter addresses some of those basic laws.

BASIC LAWS AFFECTING STUDENT RIGHTS

Most students come to college early in their adult lives. Some are barely emancipated from their parents, whereas others have been on their own for a longer period of time. They may not be aware of the laws that govern their education, and very often, unless the occasion arises, there is no need to delve into the laws governing the physical and psychological aspects of their education. Nevertheless, as a nursing faculty member it is your responsibility to be fully aware of the laws and how they impact the teaching/ learning environment.

The nursing code of ethics (provision 6) outlines the collective action necessary for the nurse to provide quality care. Students must be educated in such a manner that when they enter the workforce they are prepared to deliver the highest-quality care in the most ethical manner. Nurses must be taught to uphold the values central to nursing (i.e., human dignity, well-being, and respect for persons, health, and independence). It is essential to good nursing care that nurses possess wisdom, honesty, courage, compassion, and patience. Nursing faculty have a responsibility to nurture or challenge these values in the educational setting in preparing students for the healthcare environment.

Family Educational Rights and Privacy Act (FERPA)

In 1974, the Family Educational Rights and Privacy Act, also known as the Buckley Act, was enacted (U.S. Department of Education, n.d.a, n.d.b). This federal law protects the rights of students by maintaining the privacy of their records and guaranteeing students' access to their educational records. These records include students' biographic information, grades, letters of recommendation, disciplinary actions, and any correspondence between faculty and students.

Faculty have the responsibility to maintain accurate and complete records in a safe environment. Students can at any time have access to their records and may even ask to contribute content if they believe it will clarify any information that has been posted. In many educational institutions, students may be required to submit a written request to do so and will be granted permission within a specific period of time to review material that specifically relates to them.

Students who are dissatisfied with the findings in their records should have the opportunity to challenge the accuracy of the information. In some cases, a hearing may be held to settle any unanswered questions. In rare cases, such as situations that may be detrimental to the health and well-being of the student and/or his or her peers or where a violation may have been committed, a student's records may be shared with professors not directly related to the student or with persons outside of the university.

Faculty may release student information to parents only if the student has consented or if the student is younger than 18 years of age and is dependent on the parents. In other words, parental rights transfer to the student when he or she reaches the age of 18 years and attends a school beyond the high school level. Faculty working in an institution of higher learning need to realize the student's right to privacy now belongs to the student and not the parents. Therefore, student progress, grades, disciplinary proceedings, and other college records are the private property of the student and may not be shared with parents.

Today, when so many parents are burdened with the high costs of educating their children at colleges or universities, these parents may believe they are still entitled to know their child's progress and have access to educational records, just as they did when the child was in K–12. Parents may not realize that once their son or daughter enters an institution of higher learning, information related to that student's college experiences belongs to the student and not the parent. Therefore, when you receive a request from a student's parents to discuss the student's progress in the nursing program, you are not legally allowed to divulge any information. Some parents may be overprotective of their children and have come to be known as "helicopter parents" in the world of higher education. These parents want to know what is going on with the student's progress in the program and how they may help. Although these parents have good intentions, you may not share any student information with them without written consent from the student. For example, you cannot meet with a parent until the student has given consent, and the student has the right to be present at the meeting. If you are confronted with this situation, you should reach out to the college or university legal counsel for further information about handling the parent's request. If you do not adhere to the privacy rights of the student, the school may face litigation proceedings.

Americans with Disabilities Act (ADA)

The Americans with Disabilities Act (ADA) gives civil rights protections to students with disabilities and guarantees equal opportunity for these individuals to attend college. Colleges or universities are obligated to accommodate the disabilities of any student who is qualified for admission to the institution of higher education. Colleges or universities may reject applicants to a higher education program if the applicant's disability poses a direct threat to the health and safety of other individuals involved in the program. In the case of admission to a nursing program, if the applicant's disability (such as blindness or missing limbs) poses a threat to the safety of the patients the student will care for while in the nursing program, this applicant may be rejected from admission to the nursing program. Schools of nursing usually have written policies addressing the admission criteria for applicants with disabilities.

Title II of the ADA covers state colleges, universities, and vocational schools, and Title III of the ADA covers private colleges and vocational schools. Any schools, private or public, receiving federal dollars are covered by the regulations of the ADA and are required to make their programs accessible to persons with disabilities. Private secondary schools that do not receive federal funding are not covered under Title II of the ADA but are still required to make their schools accessible to the disabled; however, such schools are not held to the same standards as federally funded schools.

Faculty have a legal obligation to understand the laws regarding students with disabilities and the logistics of providing accommodations for these students. The ADA has provisions to protect students during their educational experience. Faculty are responsible for being aware of these provisions, and students have the responsibility to request the necessary accommodations. Note that when dealing with students you may not ask questions about their disabilities that may appear discriminatory. Also, insurance companies cannot legally refuse to insure individuals with disabilities.

In the classroom, accommodations must be made for students requiring wheelchair access, aids for various services, and enhanced ease of communication. There must be architectural access and egress for all buildings. Aside from physical disabilities, students may have learning disabilities that require accommodations to address their learning needs. In the nursing program you are more likely to encounter students with learning disabilities than physical disabilities. In these cases, special accommodations are made to help the students with disabilities have an equal opportunity to participate in and benefit from course activities. Faculty must provide classroom activities that do not discriminate against anyone with disabilities. Some challenges that faculty may face include modifying the syllabus or specific testing strategies to accommodate the student. Some possible accommodations may include adjusting due dates, providing alternative methods of test taking, and allowing note takers into the classroom. Faculty may also choose to provide a written summary of the classroom lectures and to carry out after-class meetings to clarify any subject matter that may have been missed. Faculty are not required to completely readjust the syllabus if it will fundamentally change the nature of the class. Other accommodations may include extended time for test taking, the use of hearing and visual aids, and audio/video taping of class sessions.

Most schools request written documentation of a disability, especially if the disability is hidden, such as a learning disability, mental or psychiatric disability, or other chronic impairments. The documentation is confidential and is kept in the student's permanent record. Most students are quite adept at advocating for their personal disability needs. Students with disabilities need to be registered with the Office of Specialized Services at the college or university. Once registered, these students are given the appropriate documents identifying the special accommodations they require while enrolled in school. The office will send a written communication to the faculty as to what accommodations are needed, but not necessarily what the disabilities are. Faculty are required to honor these special accommodations.

As a new faculty member, you may want to become more familiar with the policies and procedures established for meeting the educational needs of students with disabilities (U.S. Department of Justice, Civil Rights Division, n.d.). Students with hidden disabilities who do not need any accommodations may choose not to disclose them. Initial questions you need to ask regarding the ADA are: How do I locate the ADA/504 coordinator, who can help you with your possible need for accommodations? Where can I get disability awareness training? What are some of the challenges I may face when dealing with students with disabilities at this college?

F-1 STUDENT VISA ISSUES

The U.S. government added amendments to the basic Immigration and Nationality Act of 1952 after the terrorist attacks of September 11, 2001. These new regulations and procedures for admitting foreign visitors to the United States affect foreign students, teachers, and other professionals who come to the United States on student, exchange, and work visas (Department of Homeland Security, n.d.).

Foreign visitors who come to the United States to receive an education must apply for an F-1 visa through the U.S. embassy in their home country (Immigration Direct, n.d.). An F-1 visa, which is issued by the U.S. Departments of State and Homeland Security, is considered a nonimmigrant visa because it is issued to individuals who do not intend to remain in the United States after the completion of their academic studies. Therefore, F-1 visas are known as *academic student visas* and are issued for the F-1 student's attendance at one specific college or university approved by U.S. Citizenship and Immigration Services (USCIS). To apply for an F-1 student visa, the individual must have a 1-20 form issued by an approved college or university the student plans to attend. Once the 1-20 form is signed by the college or university, the individual is considered for an F-1 visa.

To obtain an F-1 visa, students must be able to meet their financial obligations to the college or university that sponsors them. This financial sponsorship varies among institutions of higher education. Students with F-1 visas must also show they are able to support themselves while in the United States attending a full-time degree or academic program because opportunities for legal employment are limited. F-1 students are not permitted to work in the United States. However, after one year of academic studies, the student may declare economic hardship and seek on-campus employment. With prior authorization from the USCIS and Homeland Security, students may work on campus and off campus in situations involving curriculum practice training; however, this employment is usually limited to 20 hours weekly. Once approved by the USCIS and Homeland Security, these students must apply for Social Security numbers. F-1 students employed in other areas not approved by the USCIS and Homeland Security are working illegally and subject to deportation.

The F-1 visa is valid for as long as it takes the student to finish a course of study while enrolled full time in a college or university approved by the USCIS. To be enrolled as a full-time student in a college or university, the F-1 student must carry at least 12 credits per semester. Occasionally exceptions to enrollment as a full-time student can be granted for medical reasons or if the student is in the last semester of study. If the F-1 student transfers to another institution of higher education, the International Office from the university or college where the student is enrolled must complete the necessary transfer papers and notify Homeland Security. Any changes in a student's

F-1 visa status must be reported immediately to Homeland Security through the Student and Exchange Visitor Information System (SEVIS).

F-1 students do not qualify for work-study programs. However, after completing an academic program of study that included a degree in science, technology, engineering, or mathematics, the USCIS may grant an extension to the employment period for these students who require continued practical training in their field of study. This employment-authorized practical training may be extended to 29 months. Once these students have completed their course of study and practical training, they have 60 days to depart from the United States.

How do these F-1 visa regulations affect the nursing students currently enrolled in the nursing program where you are a faculty member? These F-1 nursing students are in this country to obtain a nursing education degree from a two- or four-year college or university and to successfully complete the licensure examination, NCLEX-RN. At the successful completion of this program of study, F-1 nursing students may submit an application to the state board of nursing to take the licensure exam. Once the state board of nursing has received the student's application and the appropriate documents from the college or university, the student may sit for the RN licensure exam. Upon successful completion of the licensing exam, and before a license is issued to the student, the state board of nursing must receive the appropriate immigration documents from USCIS and Homeland Security and the student must apply for and obtain a Social Security number.

Once the F-1 nursing student has graduated from an approved college or university with a degree in nursing and has successfully passed the licensure examination as a registered professional nurse, he or she often hopes to obtain employment as an RN in the United States. However, to be employed as an RN in the United States, RNs with an F-1 visa must find employers that will sponsor them. If they are not able to find sponsored employment, they are expected to leave the United States and return home.

To delay their return home, RNs with F-1 visas may decide to continue their professional education in nursing. Graduates from an associate degree program may enroll in an RN to BSN program, and graduates from a generic RN program may enroll in a master's degree program. These RNs with F-1 visas are responsible for informing the USCIS and Homeland Security of their intentions to continue their education, and the 1-20 form must be completed by the college or university for the F-1 visa to remain valid.

At times, a nursing student with an F-1 visa may fail out of a nursing program. If this happens, the student may transfer to a different program of study in the same college or university or seek admission to another nursing program in a different college or university. When this happens, it is the responsibility of the student and the institution of higher education to notify the USCIS and Homeland Security of the changes. Should the student decide not to continue to pursue an education in the United States, she or he must depart the United States within 60 days.

Remember, students with F-1 visas are not here to seek citizenship and cannot apply for a green card; however, F-1 visas are good for five years, and after that time these individuals may apply for a green card provided they are sponsored by a relative who is a U.S. citizen. Individuals with a U.S. university degree have a much better chance of being granted permanent residence in the United States.

ACADEMIC GRADE GRIEVANCES

Students have the right to challenge a final course grade. This right to an academic grievance by students is usually found in the policies and procedures of the college or university and the student handbook. The procedures for students to follow when challenging the final course grade usually adhere to this general protocol:

1. The student discusses the grade dispute with the faculty member within a specified period of time following the end of the course, as designated by the college or university.
2. If the grade dispute is not resolved, the student submits a written complaint to the faculty member within a certain number of days; the faculty member must respond in writing to the student within a certain number of days.
3. If the student feels the written response from the faculty member indicates no grade change should be made, the student may then present an appeal in writing to the appropriate dean or department chair within a certain number of days.
4. The department dean or chair reviews the documentation received from the student and faculty member. At this point the department dean or chair may call for a meeting with the student and faculty member to ascertain any clarification of issues or feelings present. A written response by the dean or department chair is given to the student and faculty member within a certain number of days.
5. If the student does not agree with the decision made by the department chair or dean, the student may appeal the grade at a higher administrative level such as the academic vice president or provost within a certain number of days. The decision of the academic vice president or provost is final in the matter of the grade dispute.

When the time comes for you to issue final course grades, you will quickly realize some students are not pleased with their grade and believe they should have achieved a higher one. When this happens, you need to inform students of your availability to discuss their concerns regarding their final course grade. Keep in mind, however, the academic freedom enjoyed by faculty give only faculty the right to change a grade.

You make the decision of whether to change students' final grades; however, students have the right to appeal your decision. If your decision was not to change a student's final grade, you need to direct the student to the school's policy on grade appeal. Usually if a meeting occurs between you and the student and the student is given a complete explanation for how the grade was determined, no further action is taken by the student.

Unfortunately, there will be times when students take the appeal process all the way to higher administration. Fortunately, in most cases, higher administration supports the faculty's grade decision and respects the issuing of grades as the sole prerogative of faculty.

NURSING PROGRAM ADMISSION REQUIREMENTS

All nursing programs will have a student handbook addressing the requirements for admission and continued enrollment in the nursing program. As a faculty member, you need to become very familiar with the policies contained in this handbook. These policies outline some of your responsibilities toward students and the nursing program. In addition to containing policies related to program admission, progression through the program, and withdrawal or termination from the program, this handbook contains the following important policies having direct implications for your role as faculty.

Criminal Background Checks

In recent years, criminal background checks have become a vital requirement for students seeking admission to a nursing problem. While in a nursing program, students are engaged in patient care at different clinical agencies. To help protect the clients and patients in these agencies, state law, accreditation standards, or agency policies may require nursing students to undergo background checks. Boards of nursing encourage nursing programs and clinical agencies to work collaboratively in establishing standardized policies regarding background checks. The board of nursing recommends that the policy on background checks, like other program policies, be published in documents available to the student at the time of application to the program.

Results of the background checks are made available to the student and to the school of nursing. All background checks are treated as confidential. Any negative information gathered from the background check is subject to investigation and may prevent the applicant's admission to the nursing program. Crimes committed, usually within a seven-year time frame, that may prevent admission to a nursing program include:

- Felony convictions
- Sexual assault or rape
- Child or elder abuse

- Homicide
- Any charge related to illegal drug possession, use, or trafficking
- Assault or battery
- Misdemeanor theft or grand theft committed within a certain time period
- Embezzlement, bribery, fraud, or racketeering
- Driving under the influence (DUI) within a specific period of time
- Arson
- Kidnapping
- Forgery or counterfeiting
- Insurance fraud

Nursing programs and clinical agencies working together will review students with prior convictions on an individual basis before deciding if each student will be allowed to attend a clinical agency. If a student's background check prohibits the student from attending clinical agencies, this student cannot satisfy program requirements and may not be admitted to the nursing program. Background checks by the U.S. Department of Justice are required for all individuals seeking RN licensure in the United States.

Health Requirements

Schools of nursing have written policies regarding the health requirements of students seeking admission to the nursing program. These requirements include, but are not limited to, the following:

- Tdap (tetanus, diphtheria, and pertussis) immunization
- Tuberculin skin test by Mantoux (PPD)
- Hepatitis B seropositivity
- Varicella (chickenpox) seropositivity
- Measles seropositivity
- Rubella seropositivity
- Mumps seropositivity
- Drug screening
- Proof of health insurance

If students do not have these tests and healthcare requirements satisfied prior to admission to the program, they may forfeit admission. Once enrolled in the program, these healthcare requirements must be kept up-to-date for the students to continue clinical coursework. The nursing program should have a system in place that allows faculty to track students who are noncompliant with the healthcare requirements. Faculty cannot allow students to attend a clinical experience if these requirements are not satisfied. If students cannot attend clinical experiences as scheduled, they may be in jeopardy of failing the nursing course.

Certifications

Students who seek admission to a nursing program must be certified in cardiopulmonary resuscitation (CPR) basic life support. Certification in CPR is usually a mandatory requirement for nursing students who will be attending healthcare organizations for their clinical experience. This certification is issued by the American Heart Association and includes recognition of cardiovascular disease; infant, child, and adult CPR; one- and two-person rescue; and foreign body management. Certification must be renewed on an annual basis throughout the program. Faculty cannot allow students without a valid CPR card to care for patients in the clinical setting.

Liability Insurance

All students enrolled in a nursing program must carry their own malpractice insurance to enter the clinical agencies with which the school of nursing has contractual agreements. Each student is responsible for paying the fee for this liability insurance annually. Remember, students are responsible for their own actions in the clinical setting and are not covered under your malpractice insurance. Students who do not have liability insurance are not permitted to care for patients in any healthcare agency.

Admission Testing and Prerequisite Course Requirements

To gain admission to a nursing program, some colleges or universities require students to pass an admission test and/or provide scores from standardized tests completed prior to admission to the college or university. Most nursing programs require the student to complete certain prerequisites before entering the nursing program. These prerequisites usually include chemistry, anatomy and physiology, microbiology, and algebra. In addition to these prerequisites, students are required to complete the general education course requirements defined by the college or university granting the degree. You need to become familiar with the course catalog listing the sequence of courses required for a degree in nursing. The course catalog will describe the courses, credit allocation, prerequisites, and corequisites for each nursing course.

Traditionally, students spend each week of the semester attending didactic lectures in the classroom, laboratory experiences, and time in a clinical agency applying the knowledge they have learned to patient care using the nursing process. The amount of time allocated for these learning experiences will vary and is defined by the nursing program according to the outcome objectives for the semester. You will read more about your responsibilities in the classroom and clinical settings in future chapters of this book.

Online education has become a frequently used teaching methodology in this age of technology. Some nursing programs use online education as a means for delivering course content. Generally, online education is frequently used in nursing programs granting a BS degree to RNs as well as master's and doctoral degrees in nursing. The seven principles for good practice identified by Chickering and Gamson (1999) provide guidance for those charged with the responsibility of designing courses to be taught online. Faculty roles and responsibilities in the development and implementation of online education will be addressed in Chapter 12.

While in a nursing program, students are assigned different clinical experiences in the healthcare environment, such as acute care hospitals; rehabilitation centers; long-term care facilities; outpatient urgent centers; community settings including schools, home care, and hospice; and public health centers. Students are given this exposure to different clinical settings to learn the role of the registered nurse in these different environments. The decision to assign students to these different clinical settings will depend on the course objectives and student learning outcomes. As faculty, you are responsible for the planning and implementation of the students' experiences in these different clinical settings. This important faculty role will be addressed in Chapters 8 and 10.

ACCREDITATION IN HIGHER EDUCATION

As a practitioner who has worked in a healthcare setting, the idea of having accreditation is not a new concept to you. Healthcare accreditation ensures all practitioners and healthcare agencies have met the necessary standards of practice, competency, and ethics to ensure the delivery of quality patient care. This accreditation is a voluntary process sought by several different healthcare environments such as hospitals, ambulatory home care centers, behavioral health centers, and rehabilitation facilities, to name a few.

Colleges and universities seek accreditation as a testimony to the public that they are meeting the standards for quality education. In addition to ensuring quality education, accreditation by colleges or universities is required for access to federal funds for student aid, smooth transfer of credits among colleges and universities, and evaluation of job credentials by employers. There are numerous accrediting organizations for higher education in the United States. To ensure these accrediting organizations employ appropriate and fair practices in decision making when assessing academic quality and encouraging change or needed improvements in colleges and university programs, these accrediting organizations require recognition by the Council for Higher Education Accreditation (CHEA) and/or the U.S. Department of Education (USDE).

Council for Higher Education Accreditation (CHEA)

The Council for Higher Education Accreditation (CHEA) is a private, nonprofit national organization given the authority to affirm or deny academic legitimacy and recognition of accrediting organizations. Recognition is awarded to accrediting agencies that have met standards that advance academic quality, demonstrate accountability, encourage purposeful change and needed improvement, employ appropriate and fair procedures in decision making, continually reassess accreditation practices, and sustain fiscal stability (CHEA, n.d.a).

There are four types of accrediting organizations in the United States—regional, faith-related, career-related, and programmatic. Nursing faculty employed in a college or university need to be familiar with regional and programmatic accrediting agencies. Regional accreditation recognized by CHEA applies to public and private degree-granting two- and four-year institutions. The name of the regional accrediting organization that accredits a college or university is based on the geographic location of the institution (CHEA, n.d.c). Programmatic accreditation applies to specialized programs or schools that are part of the college or university. The name of the programmatic accrediting organization will depend on the program's area of specialization (CHEA, n.d.b).

Accreditation of institutions (regional) and programs (specialized) is cyclic and the length of accreditation may range from a few years to as many as 10 years. Accreditation is an ongoing process for colleges and universities and the specialized programs within these institutions. Periodic review is a fact of life in higher education. When institutions or programs seek accreditation, they proceed through a number of steps stipulated by the accrediting agency.

- *Self-study:* All those associated with the institution or program participate in the self-study process by evaluating the institution's or program's compliance with the standards identified by the accrediting agency. A written summary of the strengths and weaknesses is identified, along with plans for improvement. This written summary, the self-study report, is submitted to the accrediting agency for review.
- *Peer review:* The self-study report is reviewed by visiting team members from the accrediting agency in preparation for their visit to the institution or program.
- *Site visit:* Accrediting agencies send a visiting team to review the institution or program. The self-study report provides the foundation for the visit. The purpose of the visit by the team members is to evaluate, clarify, verify, and confirm information presented in the self-study report. This site visit also gives the institution or program an opportunity to demonstrate firsthand the actual practices occurring in the institution or program and for site visitors to verify congruence.
- *Site visitor's report and judgment:* Accrediting organizations have decision-making bodies (commissions) that review site visitor reports and may affirm, reaffirm, or deny accreditation. Appeals processes are also in place for institutions and programs denied accreditation.

U.S. Department of Education (USDE)

The U.S. Department of Education (USDE) does not accredit educational institutions but maintains recognition standards that institutions of higher education need to meet to qualify for federal funds for student financial aid. Recognition standards set forth by the USDE require accrediting agencies to maintain criteria related to the following:

- Student success, course completion, and job placement rates with respect to institution mission
- Curricula
- Faculty
- Facilities, equipment, and supplies
- Fiscal and administrative capacity
- Student support services
- Recruiting and admission practices, academic calendars, catalogs, grading, and advertising
- Measures of program length and the objectives of the degrees or credentials offered
- Record of student complaints
- Record of compliance with the institution's responsibilities under Title IV (federal student assistance programs) and the results of financial audits

In summary, the USDE ensures accrediting organizations contribute to maintaining and improving the academic quality of institutions and programs that receive federal funds.

NURSING PROGRAM ACCREDITATION

Two accrediting agencies used by most nursing programs throughout the United States are the Accreditation Commission for Education in Nursing (ACEN), formerly known as the National League for Nursing Accrediting Commission (NLNAC), and the Commission on Collegiate Nursing Education (CCNE). Nursing programs voluntarily seek accreditation from either of these two agencies, which ensure the program's curriculum meets the standards and criteria for educational quality and improvement in nursing education.

As nursing faculty, you will become actively involved in preparing for an accreditation review by either of these agencies. You need to be very familiar with the accreditation manual containing the standards and criteria for the type of nursing program where you are employed. Each accrediting agency has a manual specifically explaining in depth the accreditation process and procedures, the standards and criteria that are required of nursing programs, the responsibilities of the accrediting agency team members and the nursing education unit, the decision-making process for awarding accreditation, the appeal process, and time frames for reaccreditation. These accreditation manuals can be obtained on each agency's website (www.acenursing.org or www.aacn.nche.edu).

Accreditation Commission for Education in Nursing (ACEN)

The ACEN is recognized as the accrediting body for all nursing programs endorsed by the USDE, the CHEA, and the National Council of State Boards of Nursing (NCSBN). The purpose of the ACEN is to provide initial and continuing accreditation of practical nursing programs, diploma programs, associate degree programs, master's programs, post-master's certificate programs, and clinical doctorate programs. The ACEN *Standards and Criteria* manual for these various nursing programs can be found on the organization's website. The ACEN has a four-step process for evaluating nursing programs, beginning with the program's self-review and a self-study report submitted to the ACEN. After the self-study report has been submitted, the next step is a site visit by peer evaluators, who then submit a visitor's report to ACEN. The third step involves a peer evaluation review panel from the ACEN that examines the nursing program's self-study report and the site visitor's report. The final step is a decision on accreditation status by the ACEN board of commissioners.

The decision on accreditation status may confirm the nursing program's compliance with all ACEN standards, in which case the next accreditation visit will be in eight years. If this was an initial program accreditation, then the next accreditation visit will be in five years. However, if the program is noncompliant with one or two standards, the school of nursing must submit a follow-up report to the ACEN, and the next accreditation visit will be in two years with the anticipation that the program will be found compliant in all standards. Based on this follow-up report from the school of nursing and the recommendations of the evaluation review panel, a final decision regarding continued accreditation status is made by the ACEN.

Throughout the nursing school's period of accreditation, the school is required to submit an annual report to the ACEN. This annual report consists of the following information:

- Enrollment numbers
- Graduation numbers
- Faculty members and credentials
- Substantive changes made in the program
- Complaints about the program
- Job placement rates
- Licensure and certification pass rates

Commission on Collegiate Nursing Education (CCNE)

The CCNE is also a national accrediting agency recognized by the USDE that accredits nursing programs awarding a bachelor of science in nursing (BSN), graduate nursing programs, and residency programs (CCNE, n.d.). Similar to the ACEN, CCNE accreditation supports and encourages continuing self-assessment by nursing programs; however, the CCNE monitors not only nursing programs, but also the health industry to determine the core competencies required from new graduates. The CCNE has endorsed several documents developed by other organizations related to advanced practice nursing and specialty organizations. These documents identify the core competencies required by primary and acute care nurse practitioners in specialty areas such as adult, family, gerontological, and psychiatric mental health nursing.

National Council of the State Boards of Nursing (NCSBN)

The NCSBN was founded in 1978 as a nonprofit organization to bring together state boards of nursing with common interests and concerns for the health, safety, and welfare needs of the public. The NCSBN's membership includes the boards of nursing in 50 states, the District of Columbia, and four U.S. territories—Samoa, Guam, Northern Mariana Islands, and the Virgin Islands. In addition to monitoring trends in nursing practice and public policy, the NCSBN is responsible for the development of the NCLEX-RN and NCLEX-LPN licensing examinations (NCSBN, n.d.a, n.d.b).

Boards of nursing (BONs) are state government agencies responsible for the regulation of nursing practice by outlining the standards for safe practice, issuing licenses to practice nursing, monitoring licensees' compliance with state laws, and taking corrective action against nurses who have demonstrated unsafe nursing practice. Nurses from each state are expected to comply with the rules and regulations set forth in that state's Nurse Practice Act. In addition to protecting the public through regulation of nursing licensees, the BON evaluates whether the education provided by nursing programs conforms to regulatory standards of the Nurse Practice Act, thereby giving the BON jurisdiction over the regulation of nursing programs. Nursing graduates must show evidence of graduating from a BON-approved program to be eligible to take the NCLEX-RN. This oversight of nursing education programs extends the BON's legal authority to closing nursing programs that do not meet standards and have high licensure exam failure rates. Unlike the BONs, national accreditation agencies do not have the statutory authority to close a nursing program that does not meet standards. However, because the mission of the national nursing accreditation agencies is to assess the quality and effectiveness of nursing programs in the preparation of graduates who are clinically competent to practice entry-level nursing standards, program approval by these national accreditation agencies ensures the nursing program is in compliance with the BON's rules and regulations.

Most boards of nursing do not require students to graduate from nursing programs having national nursing accreditation from ACEN or CCNE to take the NCLEX-RN examination. However, as of February 2012, 96 percent of all baccalaureate or master's entry programs, 80 percent of diploma programs, 52 percent of associate degree programs, and 10 percent of practical nursing programs were nationally accredited (NCSBN, 2012a). Calls for innovation in nursing education prompted by the Institute of Medicine's *Report on the Future of Nursing Education* (2011) have sparked recommendations by the NCSBN asking all prelicensure nursing programs to be accredited by a national nursing accreditation agency recognized by the USDE by 2020. The specifics of how BONs and national accreditation agencies will collaborate to ensure safe and quality nursing care is an ongoing issue open to much deliberation and debate (www .ncsbn.org). At a time when the profession is lobbying for the advancement of nursing practice, students who graduate from a nursing program with BON accreditation but no accreditation from a national nursing accreditation agency may limit their acceptance into an advanced degree nursing program.

It is important for you to understand the roles and responsibilities of accrediting agencies and the board of nursing as well as the collegial relationships between these two groups that impact on the quality of nursing education and the future of the nursing workforce.

NCLEX-RN Examination

The NCLEX-RN examination is a nationally administered, computer adaptive testing (CAT) method that measures students' qualifications for entry-level practice in the registered nurse profession. The six-hour exam consists of 265 questions, and nurse candidates must answer a minimum of 75 questions. Question formats include multiple choice, fill-in-the-blank calculation, ordered response, and/or hot spots and may include charts, tables, graphs, sound, and video. Test questions are written at the application or higher level of cognitive ability and require more complex thought processing.

The test plan structure follows the Client Needs Framework, which is divided into four main categories. These four main categories are further divided into subcategories as follows:

- Safe and Effective Care Environment
  - Management of Care
  - Safety and Infection Control
- Health Promotion
- Psychosocial Integrity
- Physiological Integrity
  - Basic Care and Comfort
  - Pharmacological and Parenteral Therapies

- Reduction of Risk Potential
- Physiological Adaptation

Integrated throughout these Client Needs categories are the fundamental processes germane to the practice of nursing. These integrated processes as defined in the NCLEX-RN test plan are:

- *Nursing process:* This is a scientific, clinical reasoning approach to patient care involving assessment, planning, implementation, and evaluation.
- *Caring:* This is a collaborative environment where the nurse provides encouragement, hope, support, and compassion to the patient in an interactive relationship.
- *Communication and documentation:* This includes the verbal and nonverbal interactions among the nurse, patient, family, and members of the healthcare team, recorded in writing or electronically, that demonstrate adherence to standards of practice and accountability for the provision of care.
- *Teaching and learning:* This is the act of imparting knowledge and skills to patients and/or families leading to changes in behavior (NCSBN, 2012b).

A certain percentage of test questions in each of the Client Needs categories is determined by members of the NCLEX-RN examination committee. This distribution of content can be found in the NCLEX-RN test plan on the NCSBN website, as can an overview of the content included in the Client Needs categories.

Faculty need to be familiar with the content area addressed in each Client Needs category because this content needs to be included in the program's curriculum. **Table 2-1** reviews these categories and the content within each category as identified in the NCLEX-RN examination test plan.

TABLE 2-1 Safe and Effective Care Environment	
Management of Care	
• Advanced Directives	• Continuity of Care
• Advocacy	• Establishing Priorities
• Assignment, Delegation, Supervision	• Ethical Practice
• Case Management	• Informed Consent
• Client Rights	• Information Technology
• Collaboration with Interdisciplinary Team	• Legal Rights and Responsibilities
• Concepts of Management	• Performance Improvement (Quality Improvement)
• Confidentiality/Information Security	• Referrals

(continues)

TABLE 2-1 Safe and Effective Care Environment (*Continued*)

Safety and Infection Control

- Accident/Error/Injury Prevention
- Emergency Response Plan
- Ergonomic Principles
- Handling Hazardous and Infectious Materials
- Home Safety
- Reporting of Incidents/Event/Irregular Occurrence/Variance

- Safe Use of Equipment
- Security Plan
- Standard Precautions/Transmission-Based Precautions/Surgical Asepsis
- Use of Restraints/Safety Devices

Health Promotion and Maintenance

- Aging Process
- Ante/Intra/Postpartum and Newborn Care
- Developmental Stages and Transitions
- Health Promotion/Disease Prevention
- Health Screening

- High-Risk Behaviors
- Lifestyle Choices
- Self-Care
- Techniques of Physical Assessment

Psychosocial Integrity

- Abuse/Neglect
- Behavioral Interventions
- Chemical and Other Dependencies/Substance Use Disorder
- Coping Mechanisms
- Crisis Intervention
- Cultural Awareness/Cultural Influences on Health
- End-of-life Care

- Family Dynamics
- Grief and Loss
- Mental Health Concepts
- Sensory/Perceptual Alterations
- Stress Management
- Support Systems
- Therapeutic Communication
- Therapeutic Environment

Physiological Integrity

Basic Care and Comfort

- Assistive Devices
- Elimination
- Mobility/Immobility
- Nonpharmacological Comfort Interventions

- Nutrition and Oral Hydration
- Personal Hygiene
- Rest and Sleep

Pharmacological and Parenteral Therapies	
• Adverse Effects/Contraindications/Side Effects/Interactions • Blood and Blood Products • Central Venous Access Devices • Dosage Calculation	• Expected Actions/Outcomes • Parenteral/Intravenous Therapies • Pharmacological Pain Management • Total Parenteral Nutrition
Reduction of Risk Potential	
• Changes/Abnormalities in Vital Signs • Diagnostic Tests • Laboratory Values • Potential for Alterations in Body Systems • Potential for Complications of Diagnostic Tests/Treatments/Procedures	• Potential Complications from Surgical Procedures and Health Alterations • System-Specific Assessments • Therapeutic Procedures
Physiological Adaptation	
• Alterations in Body Systems • Fluid and Electrolyte Imbalances • Hemodynamics • Illness Management	• Medical Emergencies • Pathophysiology • Unexpected Response to Therapies
Modified from National Council of State Boards of Nursing. (2012). NCLEX-RN® Examination. Retrieved from https://www.ncsbn.org/2013_NCLEX_RN_Test_Plan.pdf.	

Faculty need to be familiar with these Client Needs categories and the integrated process applied throughout the Client Needs categories because these should serve as a blueprint for when you develop test questions within a course.

CASE STUDIES

1. You have a student who is presently failing your pediatric nursing course. His mother has sent you an email asking to meet with you at your earliest convenience to discuss her son's progress in your course. How would you handle this situation under the FERPA law?
2. A student who qualifies for ADA accommodations and is in your medical–surgical nursing course has informed you that she needs extra time to take the exam next week. How would you handle this situation, following the ADA regulations?
3. A student with an F-1 education visa has failed your course. What advice would you give this student regarding the process he needs to follow to remain enrolled at this college and possibly return to the nursing program?

4. A student is unhappy with the final grade he has received in your nursing course. How would you handle this situation, and what advice would you give this student regarding his student rights in academia?
5. You are working in the advising center at your college, and a student approaches you for advice on the admission requirements for the nursing program. How would you respond to this student?
6. Explain the accreditation process followed by your school of nursing.
7. You are orienting your nursing students to the format of the NCLEX-RN test plan. Explain how this test is constructed to evaluate students' ability to function as a beginning licensed practitioner.

REFERENCES

Chickering, A. W., Gamson, Z. F. (1999). Development and adaptations of the seven principles for good practice in undergraduate education. *New Directions for Teaching and Learning, 1999*(80), 75–81.

Commission on Collegiate Nursing Education (CCNE). (n.d.). CCNE accreditation. Retrieved from http://www.aacn.nche.edu/ccne-accreditation

Council for Higher Education Accreditation (CHEA). (n.d.a). Homepage. Retrieved from http://chea.org

Council for Higher Education Accreditation (CHEA). (n.d.b). Programmatic accrediting organizations 2015–2016. Retrieved from http://www.chea.org/Directories/special.asp

Council for Higher Education Accreditation (CHEA). (n.d.c). Regional accrediting organizations 2015–2016. Retrieved from http://www.chea.org/Directories/regional.asp

Immigration Direct. (n.d.). Apply for a U.S. F-1 student visa. Retrieved from https://www.immigrationdirect.com/visas/student/F-1-Visa.jsp

Institute of Medicine. (2010). *The future of nursing: Leading change, advancing health*. Washington, DC: National Academies of Health.

National Council of State Boards of Nursing (NCSBN). (2012a). A preferred future for prelicensure program approval: Part II. Strategies for moving forward. Retrieved from https://www.ncsbn.org/A_Preferred_Future_for_Prelicensure_Program_PartII_wAppendices2012.pdf

National Council of State Boards of Nursing. (2012b). NCLEX-RN® Examination. Retrieved from https://www.ncsbn.org/2013_NCLEX_RN_Test_Plan.pdf

National Council of State Boards of Nursing (NCSBN). (n.d.a). Home page. Retrieved from http://www.ncsbn.org

National Council of State Boards of Nursing (NCSBN). (n.d.b). NCLEX & other exams. Retrieved from https://www.ncsbn.org/nclex.htm

U.S. Department of Education (USDE). (n.d.a). Family Educational Rights and Privacy Act (FERPA). Retrieved from http://www2.ed.gov/policy/gen/guid/fpco/ferpa/index.html

U.S. Department of Education (USDE). (n.d.b). Homepage. Retrieved from http://www.ed.gov

U.S. Department of Homeland Security. (n.d.). Students and employment. Retrieved from https://www.uscis.gov/working-united-states/students-and-exchange-visitors/students-and-employment

U.S. Department of Justice, Civil Rights Division. (n.d.). Information and technical assistance on the Americans with Disabilities Act. Retrieved from http://www.ada.gov

Classroom Teaching

CHAPTER 3

Curriculum Development

OBJECTIVES

- Define curriculum development.
- Analyze the components of a nursing curriculum.
- Determine appropriate curricula designs based on educational levels.
- Analyze a curriculum case study in preparation for taking on a new faculty role.

As you think about taking on the role of nursing educator, there are some important factors to consider. Before applying for the job, you should explore several institutes of higher education to see which types of programs are being offered. Next, you should explore whether there is an option to teach your preferred subjects at either the associate, baccalaureate, or master's levels. It is not unusual for some new faculty to start by teaching at the associate-degree level, so as to gain confidence in the classroom. Once they become comfortable, they go on to teach at the baccalaureate level and later progress to teaching at the graduate level. Other considerations may include the discipline/content to be taught and one's ability to do so, and the availability of promotion and advancement opportunities within the organization.

Whatever your preferences, one of the major roles of faculty that you will encounter is developing and implementing the curriculum. As a new faculty member you may initially be more concerned with honing your teaching skills and managing the classroom environment, and pay little attention to the overall process of curriculum development. However, once you have delved into the full faculty role, not only will you be expected to understand the process of curriculum development, but you also may find yourself involved as a member of a curriculum development team. By becoming a member of this important team you will be exposed to a deeper understanding of the entire process and its impact on the nursing program. Once you gain an intimate understanding of curriculum development, it will become clear to you how constructs are developed, goals and objectives established, and outcomes measured and evaluated. Furthermore, you will have a clear understanding of why it is necessary to periodically redesign the curriculum to meet changes in societal needs.

DEFINING CURRICULUM DEVELOPMENT

This chapter starts by establishing a grounded definition for curriculum development. It goes on to describe components of a curriculum, discuss factors influencing curriculum development, describe steps in choosing a curriculum design, and outline challenges to curriculum development.

The literature is replete with definitions of the word *curriculum*; it is therefore important for us to establish consistency in the way we use this word throughout this text. A curriculum is an academic plan or course of study that clearly lays out goals for student learning, the content to be learned, the sequence in which material will be taught, the methods of instructions, the teaching resources to be used, who will be responsible for carrying out the teaching, and how the learning outcomes will be measured. It is expected that after completing the course of study, students will have gained the knowledge, skills, and attitudes that are expected within the profession.

As previously mentioned, several disciplines have designed their own definitions of curriculum, so as you explore the literature you will come across a variety of approaches to curriculum development and implementation. Even so, you will notice that curricula basically result in the same end goal of providing a program of study aimed at assisting students to attain their educational goals. The core of all nursing education programs can be linked to the type of curriculum. The curriculum forms the foundation on which all aspects of the educational program are built; it consists of a mission or vision that is congruent with that of the parent organization, a philosophy, an organizing framework, constructs, goals of the program, and course objectives.

Faculty and other responsible parties are in charge of developing and implementing the curriculum using professional nursing standards as a guide. It is extremely important that all participants in the development of the curriculum be made aware of the expected outcomes and how they will be measured. There must also be a clear understanding of the steps or learning processes that will be undertaken to ensure and measure that the outcomes are met.

The teacher, students, resources, and educational environment are the major factors in the success of the learning process. Dillon (2009) describes the teacher as the most influential person in the teaching/learning process, one who has all the personal characteristics, qualifications, training, education, and background to make a difference in the student's learning outcomes. The student who wants to learn comes to the teaching/learning environment to gain guidance and education to help meet personal educational goals. The subject content included in the curriculum will depend greatly on the discipline of study. The method of presentation will influence the teaching/learning approach. The teaching/learning environment plays a major part in the learning process and should never be overlooked, whether it involves teaching face to face in a single classroom, online, within a community, or to society in general.

Overall, the curriculum process, design, and implementation involves a teacher, students, the subject matter to be taught, an environment in which teaching will occur, resources and methodologies, activities, expected outcomes, and methods of evaluation.

STEPS IN DEVELOPING THE CURRICULUM

Educators preparing to develop or revise a curriculum should follow steps similar to those in the familiar nursing/learning process, which include assessing, planning, developing, implementing, and evaluation.

- Start by convening a group of faculty to discuss trends, assess the needs of the organization/school, identify the content to be taught and all needed resources, and determine which environment and mode are best to deliver the specific curriculum.
- Develop a timeline and sequencing for the implementation of the curriculum and decide on measuring tools with which to evaluate the outcomes.
- The next step deals with articulating the findings and developing the curriculum. In this phase, faculty explore various philosophies and come up with a decision as to the one that best suits the organization.
- Courses are identified, and resources to assist with the implementation of the curriculum and measurements to determine student progress are decided upon.
- During the implementation phase, the program is put into practice; thereafter it is evaluated as to how well outcomes have been met.
- The information gained from formative and summative evaluations of the curriculum is used to update and redesign future programs.

Although experienced faculty are usually the first to be called on to be engaged in developing the curriculum, newer faculty have a great deal to contribute. It may seem bold to say, but some newer faculty have been exposed to more current teaching strategies, have been exposed to more current material, understand the theory of integration of technology into the curriculum, and may be more familiar with younger students' needs. Understanding the different generations of learners will be discussed in Chapter 12.

Curricular content will depend greatly on the discipline. For example, a nurse practitioner (NP) curriculum would contain mostly a higher level of content and the delivery approach would focus more on providing information that would assist the NP in assessing and prescribing. The RN curriculum, in contrast, would be geared toward providing information that will help students assess and identify situations, implement within their scope of practice, and/or report to the medical team. Once the decision has been made as to which courses will be included in the curriculum, faculty can focus on the content to be included and the types of resources needed to deliver the teaching. This information is provided in the form of a curriculum guide, which includes the mission goals and philosophy of the program, sequencing and leveling of courses, expected course outcomes, course objectives, yearly course plan, and an assessment plan. See **Appendix 3-A** for a sample course outline.

Getting Ready to Redesign the Curriculum

Prior to participating in the design and/or redesign of the curriculum, faculty will benefit from reviewing Bloom's taxonomy (see **Figure 3-1** and **Table 3-1**). Bloom's taxonomy promotes higher-order thinking in education. It is one of the most commonly used tools adopted by faculty in the design of curriculum. The taxonomy forms a structure from the simple to the complex in terms of cognitive process. For a discussion of this taxonomy, which is considered a classic in the educational literature, go to www .bloomstaxonomy.org.

Bloom's taxonomy divides the way people learn into three domains or categories: cognitive, affective, and psychomotor. Cognitive refers to knowledge or mental skills, affective refers to change in attitude or feeling, and psychomotor refers to manual or

FIGURE 3-1 Cognitive levels as stated by Bloom.

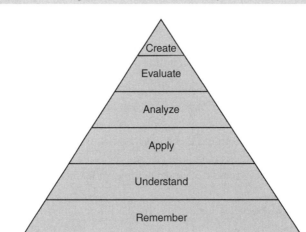

Modified from Anderson, L. W., Krathwhol, D. R., Airasian, P. W., Cruikshank, K. A., Mayer, R. E., Pintrich, P. R., . . . Wittrock, M. C. (2001). *A taxonomy for learning, teaching, and assessing: A revision of Bloom's taxonomy of educational objectives, complete edition.* Upper Saddle River, NJ: Pearson.

TABLE 3-1 Bloom's Categories with Accompanying Objectives and Statements

Category	Remember	Understand	Apply	Evaluate	Create
Objectives	List and describe	Classify and calculate	Explain and differentiate	Assess and conclude	Plan and compare
Statements	Recall basic pharmacology facts regarding medicating children.	Determine in which situations it would be most important to administer Narcan.	Explain why understanding EKG tracing is vital in monitoring a cardiac patient.	Conclude why the intra-abdominal route is best for administering insulin.	Develop a research proposal on current evidence in healthcare delivery.

physical skills. These learning behaviors can be considered as the goals of the learning process. In an orderly fashion, learners should acquire changes in their knowledge, skills, and attitude.

Hallmarks of a Good Curriculum

The National League for Nursing outlines the criteria for an appropriate curriculum (see www.nln.org). After having reviewed the hallmarks of an appropriate curriculum, you will be prepared to participate in building a curriculum that is flexible, evidence based, culturally aware, values forming, and innovative.

Components of a Curriculum: The Mission

A traditional curriculum is composed of a mission, a philosophy, constructs, goals, and objectives. No matter the method of curriculum delivery, all curricula possess some basic characteristics. The curriculum generally begins with a **mission statement**, which clearly outlines the specific services of the organization and what the program has to offer. Additionally, a mission identifies the goal of the organization, the geographic location of the target population, and the standards to which the organization holds itself.

An example of a school's mission could be as follows:

BLU Nursing Program is committed to providing quality baccalaureate and master's-level education. The mission is congruent with that of the college, with a strong emphasis on an interdisciplinary curriculum enhanced by experiential opportunities and intercultural understanding.

Graduates of the nursing programs will function in a variety of settings caring for individuals of diverse backgrounds, having been well equipped to form partnerships with professionals from other disciplines (Modified from Ramapo College of New Jersey [RCNJ] Nursing Programs, 2014).

Establishing a Philosophical Foundation for the Curriculum

As you explore information on nursing curricula, you will notice that most curricula start with the philosophy of the nursing program. The philosophy highlights the beliefs of faculty about what a nursing education ought to be and is influenced by professional nursing standards as well as the mission of the school or college. There are several educational theories and philosophies, discussion of which is outside the scope of this text; however, you may note that some nursing philosophies are developed based on the structural hierarchy of contemporary nursing knowledge. Jacqueline Fawcett (1995) developed four basic metaparadigms of nursing that serve as the underpinning to the entire universal conceptual framework for the nursing profession. According to this theory, contemporary nursing knowledge takes the form of a hierarchy, as outlined here:

- Metaparadigm concept, which sets the boundaries of the discipline and includes the roles of person, nursing, environment, and health.
- Philosophy or beliefs and values held by members of the discipline. These may be psychological or sociological.
- Conceptual models/constructs, which are abstract representations of reality. These are often referred to as organizing frameworks.
- Nursing theories, which are less abstract and more concrete than conceptual models and may vary in scope.
- Empirical indicators, which are tools used to measure theories and outcomes.

The philosophy of the program declares why certain areas are being addressed, the beliefs of the faculty regarding the areas being addressed, how education is implemented, and the recipients' expected outcomes. The philosophy springs from and is congruent with the mission of the parent organization and highlights faculty's knowledge, beliefs, and commitments to the curriculum. The philosophy also states the expectations for students who complete the program.

Constructs

Schools often develop constructs or concepts around which their curriculum is focused. This is referred to as the program's *organizing framework*. Constructs may be determined by the mission of the offerings or may be guided by competencies set forth by accrediting agencies such as the AACN, CNEA, ACEN, and other professional bodies. These agencies create guiding principles for professional nursing with the aims of protecting the public and safeguarding the welfare of customers. Common examples of constructs utilized by some nursing programs are outlined in **Table 3-2**, which contains sample objectives and potential assignments to meet these objectives. These constructs include knowledge, research and evidence base, leadership, technology, social advocacy, global issues, diversity, and role function, among others. Constructs are leveled based on students' expected outcomes at different stages of the curriculum. See **Appendix 3-B** for sample of leveled constructs.

TABLE 3-2 Sample Concepts with Matching Objectives and Applicable Assignments

Constructs	Course Objectives	Assignment
Knowledge	Apply knowledge synthesized from nursing science, basic science, social science, humanities, and educational theory to support the educator in the institution of higher learning.	Complete weekly graded written assignments on a variety of topics based on science and the humanities.
Research and evidence base	Demonstrate ability to carry out a clinical or educational evidence-based project.	Research the literature, collect data, and develop an evidence-based project on assigned units.
Technology/ information management	Utilize outcomes from a systematic plan of evaluation to suggest improvements to the teaching/learning environment.	Complete a systematic plan of evaluation on an assigned organization and make recommendations for changes.
Leadership	Analyze attributes of leadership required for a successful educator role.	Observe clinical faculty on site and assist in supervising nursing students. Model professional behaviors for students.
Role function	Function in the role of educator in an institution of higher learning. Function in the role of educator in healthcare institutions.	Collaborate with preceptor to develop and carry out a teaching plan. Teach two face-to-face classes. Make a mini-presentation to staff colleagues, faculty, and students. Participate in interdisciplinary efforts to address healthcare needs locally, regionally, nationally, and internationally.

Modified from Ramapo College of New Jersey MSN Program. (2015).

Once the program constructs have been decided upon, all objectives and course outcomes are based on these general concepts. Faculty will go on to develop the components of the curriculum outlining the role that different individuals will play in its implementation. Nursing school graduates are expected to have demonstrated competency in all outcomes.

Choosing a Curriculum Design

Designing a curriculum is a process or way of thinking or organizing disciplines and identifying content and concepts that students are expected to learn or understand during a specific period of time. It involves a broad picture of activities that students are supposed to cover during a specific program of study. Several factors need to be taken into consideration when choosing a curriculum design. Important factors include the mission and type of program, the types of students the program will attract, available resources, the environment in which the program will be carried out, and the level of administrative support. Nursing curriculum design would incorporate all the required and recommended courses that a student should complete prior to graduating from the program.

Often schools form a committee to identify which curriculum design best suits the particular organization. Faculty then vote to approve the one that is acceptable to all.

A curriculum design may be content based (i.e., organized in a traditional format that is discipline specific, such as medical–surgical or pediatric nursing) or it may be concept based (i.e., certain concepts are chosen by faculty to be addressed at different stages across the lifespan). A variety of common curriculum designs are listed in **Table 3-3**. This topic will be discussed throughout the text.

Developing Goals

Once faculty choose a curriculum design, the next step is developing goals for the curriculum. The **goals** are based on the constructs and the overall expected outcomes of the program. Goals are broad and overarching, measurable, attainable, realistic, and time bound. Program and course goals are developed with certain factors in mind, including the types of students, the clients to be served, and the type of content required for the discipline.

Developing Objectives

The course **objectives** provide a step-by-step approach on how the course goals are to be met. Although linked directly to the content, the objectives are also guided by the basic constructs of the program. Objectives are measurable and provide the framework for summative and formative evaluations. The objectives form a guide for the teacher as to which material is to be covered and a guide to the student as far as what needs to

TABLE 3-3 Some Commonly Used Curriculum Designs	
Curriculum Design	**Description**
Oregon Consortium for Nursing Education model (OCNE)	Developed in 2001 in response to the critical nursing shortage. It is a shared partnership among eight community colleges and five campuses of the Oregon Health & Science University School of Nursing. This model provides opportunities for greater numbers of students to obtain necessary clinical experiences in community-based and long-term care facilities (OCNE, 2013). Details about this program can be reviewed at www.ocne.org.
Evidence-based curriculum model	In this model, research data are used to drive the implementation of the curriculum. Learning experiences are designed to support evidence-based practice, provide a multidisciplinary approach to care, provide expertise in specialty roles, and support student clinical competency. More information on this model can be obtained at www.nln.org or www.ncsbn.org.
Competency- or outcomes-based model	Often referred to as Quality and Safety Education for Nurses (QSEN), this model was developed to provide nursing faculty with strategies to integrate quality and safety into nursing curricula. The six competencies are patient-centered care, teamwork and collaboration, evidence-based practice, quality improvement, safety, and informatics (QSEN, 2013). The scope of the curriculum focuses on the knowledge, skills, and abilities (KSAs) that embody professional nursing practice. More information can be obtained by going to www.qsen.org.
Concept-based curriculum model	Students are taught from a series of chosen concepts that are linked to evidence-based exemplars. Concepts may be chosen across the lifespan, across the environment, or along the health–illness continuum (Ebner & Hubbard, 2010).
Curriculum mapping	This design offers a framework of teaching that provides transparency into all aspects of the curriculum. In this style of delivery, teachers' work can be tracked and students have access to the entire scope of the curriculum. Most importantly, the curriculum is aligned to the program objectives in such a way that gaps in teaching can easily be identified and remedied.

be learned to meet the course outcomes as well as what will be evaluated. Faculty are required to revisit the objectives regularly as they give assignments and perform evaluation/testing. A frequent question one should ask is, "Have I provided students with enough or the right information so they can meet the stated objectives of the course?" The following is an example of a course objective with accompanying assignment:

> Analyze a variety of approaches to curriculum development using current evidence. **Assignment:** Participate in weekly discussions and analysis of relevant educational advancement and research.

The **course content** to be covered is included in the syllabus. There should be dates and timelines showing when each set of content will be covered. Content may include readings from assigned texts or other material, web searches, and independent reading assignments. Reading material may be listed as required or as recommended. Required content should relate directly to the course objectives. Recommended content may be indirectly related to the objectives but provides extra information to broaden the student's knowledge base. Content should be chosen for its relevance to the course, currency, accuracy, and overall global appeal. Assignments should assist students in meeting course outcomes.

Implementing the Curriculum Through Specific Course Syllabi

Courses that make up the curriculum are delivered via individual syllabi. The **syllabus** is essentially the working paper for each course and is a reflection of the overall program curriculum. The syllabus contains goals and objectives, expected outcomes and evaluative measures, reading requirements, a weekly content outline, and policies specific to that particular course. (See **Table 3-4** for a sample syllabus outline.) General policies are usually relegated to the student handbook. Specific policies may include those on plagiarism, class participation, class behavior, and students having special needs. At the beginning of the semester, students and faculty discuss the content of the syllabus, and the overall expectations of the course are outlined. Students are informed of the methods that will be used to perform not only the students' formative evaluations, but also their summative evaluations of the course. Once the syllabus has been reviewed and presented to the class, it is important to avoid making any changes unless they are fully presented and agreed upon by the class. If changes have to be made, they should not affect students' grades for the worse.

PROGRAM DELIVERY FORMAT

The format in which the program is to be delivered is also of utmost importance. The method of presentation will influence the teaching/learning approach. The teaching/

TABLE 3-4 Sample Syllabus Outline: Bachelor of Science in Nursing	
COURSE SYLLABUS	
Course Number:	NURS3102
Course Title:	Fundamentals of Nursing Research
Course Credit:	3 credits
Course Level:	Third Year
Prerequisite Courses:	Theoretical Basis of Nursing
	Statistics for Social Sciences
Faculty:	Faculty name
	Office phone:
	Web-enhanced class
Office Hours:	Mondays & Wednesdays 2–4 PM
Contact Hours:	14 weeks of lecture
Course Description:	
Course Goals:	
Course Objectives: *Linked to constructs*	
Teaching Methods: *Mode of delivery*	
Evaluation Methods: *How objectives will be measured*	
Required Text(s): *Primary text*	
Recommended Text(s):	
Course Requirements:	
Course Grades:	
Course Policies: *May include student expectations, academic misconduct, tardiness, or ethics*	

learning environment plays a major part in the learning process and should never be overlooked, whether it involves teaching face to face (F2F) in a single classroom, online, in a community, or to society in general.

Delivery formats may include the traditional face-to-face meeting in a classroom; a partially web-enhanced format, called hybrid; or totally online. The mode of delivery may impact to some degree the level of interaction; however, the basic content should be designed so that the educational goals can be fully achieved.

Traditional Delivery

Despite discussions to the contrary, the traditional face-to-face classroom delivery method is still very attractive to many students, especially those who may not be self-disciplined or self-motivated to do the work on their own time. According to

Petrina (1998), this type of curriculum delivery mode may be carried out in a transmissive, transactive, or transformative manner. In the transmissive orientation, information is passed from teacher to student. In the transactive method, information is discussed and negotiated between teacher and student. In the transformative method, the teacher provides content and acts more as a coach and guide for students as they decipher and learn. Flipping the classroom, discussed in Chapter 4, is one way to deliver the curriculum in a transactive manner.

Online Delivery

For returning students with multiple and sometimes competing life activities, an online design may be very attractive. This method of delivery allows students to participate in their education on their own time. Students register for courses and are oriented to an electronic platform through which the course is being delivered. A program of study is designed that allows students to participate at their own pace. There are pros and cons to this delivery method, as discussed in Chapter 4.

Hybrid Delivery

Even more appealing to some students are the web-enhanced methods of delivery. In this design, students attend face-to-face meetings at predetermined times during the semester and carry out the rest of the class via online assignments and discussions. These methods and designs will be discussed in detail in Chapter 4.

The discipline of nursing requires some form of student clinical experience to be included and accounted for in the curriculum. Students may be assigned clinical instructors to attend clinical sites, which may be supplemented with experiences of laboratory simulations. Laboratory simulations have come into favor over the last decade and are currently being used in most nursing school programs. Simulation pros and con are discussed further in Chapter 12.

INTERNAL AND EXTERNAL FACTORS AFFECTING CURRICULUM DEVELOPMENT

Designing and redesigning curricula seems to be a constant in the life of faculty. Historically, curricula have been changed and redesigned based on societal needs, political involvement, industrial and economic needs, and changing demographics. One point is constant: Curricula are not static, but rather must adjust to and be reflective of changing needs. Additionally, curricula do not undergo rapid changes; therefore, implementation must be carefully developed to ensure that all aspects of need, content, and learning outcomes have been considered.

A recent example of the need for curricular change has been the rapid and exponential growth of technology and the need to integrate technology into the curriculum. Another current reason for redesigning the curriculum, according to Keating (2010), is healthcare reform legislation, such as the Patient Protection and Affordable Care Act. Accreditation of programs by national organizations also places great responsibility on institutions to design and redesign programs that are current and flexible.

Despite the fact that nurse educators are usually held accountable for developing the curriculum, their efforts are not carried out independent of important internal and external influences. When planning to develop a new curriculum or to restructure an existing one, it is important to collaborate with stakeholders including faculty, students, administration, and consumers in the local community.

Table 3-5 summarizes the three types of factors that exert the greatest influence on curricular changes: internal, external, and organizational influences.

Internal influences on curriculum development include the mission and vision of the parent organization, the school philosophy, the quality of the program, the qualifications of the educators, the organizational management (such as directors, CEOs, presidents, and provosts), and students. Curricula are developed to reflect the college or university's mission; for example, a college that serves a small community may develop programs that will graduate students with skills that are needed in the community and would attract students from the community who want to obtain these skills. A large state college or university, in contrast, would likely develop multiple programs within the school to attract a wider, more global audience. Required faculty educational backgrounds also differ from school to school and from program to program.

TABLE 3-5 Factors Influencing Curriculum Development

Internal Factors	External Factors	Organizational Factors
Quality of faculty	Society	Organization mission
Academic discipline	Politics	Student demands
Students	Government	Resources
Program mission/vision	Stakeholders	Academic plan
Program resources	Professional associations	Leadership goals
Diversity of population	Employers	Structural availability
Quality of program	Alumni	
	Technology	
	Accrediting agencies	
	NCLEX pass rate	
	Globalization	

An aspiring educator with an MSN degree may be able to secure employment on the nursing faculty in a community college. In most cases, however, you would need to have a doctoral degree to teach at the BSN level, and definitely at the master's level in most schools. If your highest educational level is an MSN, you should continue your education so you will be prepared to teach at a higher level. If you want to carry out educational research, you will need to be doctorally prepared and should seek employment in organizations that are research focused.

Other internal forces may be related to the increased **diversity** of the population and changes in the demographics of healthcare providers. There is no doubt that over the past several years the population has become more diverse in terms of ethnicity, disability, and many other factors. Not only is the general population more diverse, but also nursing faculty and students. Nursing programs are currently developing more flexible curricula to address these rapid changes. It is important that nurses become well equipped to address the needs of the changing population. Changes in societal behavior such as increased violence in schools, increasing bioterrorism, technological advancements, new diseases such as human immunodeficiency virus (HIV) and Ebola virus, and the increasing incidence of malaria in the United States are just a few of the issues that faculty need to take into consideration when redesigning the curriculum. As previously mentioned, nurses themselves also reflect the changing population, and as such curricula must adjust to their demographics. McGuire and Scott (2006) sum up the need for addressing diversity in educational curricula by stating that an instructional paradigm shift is forcing instructional access to change from accommodation to full inclusion.

Whereas **internal influences** are linked to the needs and expectations of the faculty, administrators, students' characteristics, academic discipline, types of programs, and the resources needed to run those programs, **external forces** include the community's needs, government involvement, changing societal needs, and the need to take progress into account, such as implementing technology into programs.

To a new faculty member, it may seem farfetched that politics should have much influence on the development of a nursing program's curriculum; however, politics often exerts a major influence because the political machine is often responsible for funding schools' buildings, resources, and human resources. Along with political influences, external forces often involve stakeholders who demand that colleges prepare students to meet industry needs. Currently there is a great demand for experts in the technology and business fields. It is likely that stakeholders have begun demanding that curricula be developed to address these needs. Nurses must be adept at working in a technology-rich environment, be prepared to work in the community, and be ready to work with the aged and diverse populations. Despite the popular belief that external forces more strongly influence vocational than traditional curricula, more recently traditional curricula have come under scrutiny and under the influence of stakeholders outside of the organization.

Organizational influences on curriculum development include administrative goals and objectives, the academic plan, students' demands, structural availability, and resources. Often the curriculum will be expanded or shrunk to accommodate programs. An example of this is what is currently occurring in the nursing field: Owing to the shortage of nursing faculty, many nursing programs have decreased their student nurse enrollment due to insufficient numbers of instructors. Sometimes organizational influences may even be linked to the head administrator's personal trajectory or to the unavailability of adequate physical structures and other resources to accommodate large numbers of students.

CHALLENGES IN CURRICULUM DEVELOPMENT

Curriculum restructuring may sometimes be related to other interorganizational processes, such as long delays in obtaining committee approvals for curriculum changes due to a large amount of hierarchical bureaucracy. Accrediting organizations also set standards that influence the way the curriculum is implemented. Some of these standards bring about barriers, as noted in Keating (2010). These barriers may include accreditation standard requirements, state laws and regulations, and state-by-state approval of programs, which dictate institutional eligibility to receive financial aid.

A common phrase you may often hear is "Faculty own the curriculum." This may be true to a point, because faculty are indeed accountable for assessing, planning, implementing, and evaluating the curriculum. Faculty are challenged to properly develop a curriculum that is relevant so that students will be able to reach their academic goals. They must design flexible curricula that deliver the best educational opportunities for their students. Another important challenge lies in the fact that institutions are constantly changing and redefining themselves to keep up with healthcare trends and demands. The healthcare environments have become more diversified, with care now being delivered in ambulatory care settings and even in supermarkets. Healthcare costs have increased, and alternative approaches to delivery of care are no longer uncommon. The nursing curriculum must not only reflect these changes, but also be innovative and creative as well as appropriate to meet accreditation standards. Faculty are constantly trying to make the curriculum attractive, and nursing schools are always making changes to attract potential students. These changes sometimes focus on altering the number of credits in the program, redistributing course grade requirements, and designing curricula that are more flexible and student friendly.

In the face of the recent technology explosion, faculty are challenged to make the curriculum more interactive and less boring. Students have as much access to new and current information as faculty; therefore, faculty must sharpen their creative skills as they guide students to fulfill course requirements and meet their goals.

Iwasiw et al. (2014) sum up the issue well by stating, "Curriculum development in nursing education is a scholarly and creative process intended to produce an evidence-informed, context-relevant, unified nursing curriculum." The curriculum must be relevant, flexible, accommodating of diversity, innovative, creative, and technology infused. Organizing a curriculum not only requires faculty, evaluations, ongoing appraisals, and implementations, but also experts, community, and evidence-based practice—and the end result must align with the parent institution's framework (Keating, 2011).

Evaluation is one of the most important aspects of a curriculum. Several aspects of the curriculum must be considered. The goal must be appropriate to the program, the objectives must address the needs of the goal, and the assignments must be congruent with the objectives. Most importantly, the content must be delivered in such a way as to provide students with adequate information so that they are able to meet the expected outcomes of the program. Evaluations are done formatively and summatively. Chapter 6 focuses on curriculum evaluation, including sample tools and directions regarding evaluation techniques. Chapter 6 explores program evaluation, peer evaluation, and student evaluation.

CASE STUDY

As a nurse about to embark on a teaching career, you are currently interviewing at several schools of nursing, but you are unsure as to which questions you should ask. Having discussed this with several experienced educators, you decide to start by researching the schools to obtain a clear picture of what is involved in their program curricula, what makes up the curricula, what some challenges are at each school, and what the schools' expectations are. You decide to ask questions about the roles and responsibilities you will have to take on regarding developing the curriculum. You also have an interest in who should be responsible for developing the curriculum. You are concerned about how curriculum outcomes will be measured.

DISCUSSION QUESTIONS

1. What are some factors to consider when choosing a specific program curriculum?
2. Discuss specific issues to be taken into consideration when developing curricular frameworks.
3. Describe the main components of an official program guide.
4. List some internal factors that affect the development of a curriculum.

5. List some external factors that affect the development of a curriculum.
6. To what extent will the increased use of technology impact the development of the curriculum?
7. Explain why regulatory bodies have a great deal of influence on the development of the curriculum.
8. Discuss some crucial factors that should dictate changes and adjustments made to a curriculum.
9. Describe common strategies that faculty use to promote critical thinking in their students.
10. To what extent should faculty involve students in curriculum development?

REFERENCES

Dillon, J. T. (2009). The questions of curriculum. *Journal of Curriculum Studies, 41*(3), 343–359. doi:10.1080/00220270802433261. Retrieved from http://web.ebscohost.com/ehost/pdfviewer/pdfviewer?sid=deb50a82-6827-4cb3-8961-80f132569edb%40sessionmgr110&vid=1&hid=108

Ebner, M. K., & Hubbard, A. (2010). Concept-based learning. Community College Baccalaureate Association. Retrieved from http://www.accbd.org/wp-content/uploads/2010/08/Concept-Based-Learning-by-M.-Kathleen-Ebener-PhD-RN-and-Ann-Hubbard-Ed.D.-CNE.pdf

Fawcett, J. (1995). *Analysis and evaluation of contemporary nursing knowledge: Nursing models and theory*. Philadelphia, PA: FA Davis.

Iwasiw, C., Goldenberg, D., & Andrusyszyn, M. (2014). *Curriculum development in nursing education*. Burlington, MA: Jones & Bartlett Learning.

Keating, S. (2010). *Curriculum development and evaluation in nursing*. New York, NY: Springer.

Keating, S. (2011). *Curriculum development and evaluation in nursing* (2nd ed.). New York, NY: Springer.

McGuire, J. M., & Scott, S. S. (2006). Universal design for instruction: Extending the universal design paradigm to college instruction. *Journal of Postsecondary Education and Disability, 19*(2), 124–134.

Oregon Consortium for Nursing Education. (2013). OCNE: Curriculum. Retrieved from http://www.ocne.org/students/Curriculum.html

Petrina, S. (1998). Chapter 9: Curriculum and instructional design. Retrieved from http://www.uw-platt.edu/~steck/Petrina%20Text/Chapter%209.pdf

QSEN Institute. (2013). Competencies. Retrieved from http://qsen.org/competencies

Ramapo College of New Jersey-Nursing Programs. Constructs with course objectives and assignments

Bachelor of Science in Nursing Course Outline

Course	Course Credits	Theory/ Lecture Credits	Clinical/Lab Credits
GENERAL EDUCATION COURSES			
Anatomy and Physiology I	3	4	2
Anatomy and Physiology II	3	4	2
Microbiology I	3	2	1
Nutrition	3		
Microbiology II	3	2	1
Inorganic Chemistry	3	2	1
Statistics	3		
English II	3		
Psychology I	3		
Sociology	3		
Psychology II	3		
Intermediate Algebra	3		
Technology in Health Sciences	3		
ELECTIVE COURSES			
Modern American Literature	4		
History of Music or History of Art	3		
Cultural Diversity	3		
English or Spanish or French Studies	3		
TOTAL GEN. ED. CREDITS	**52**		
MAJOR NURSING COURSES			
Fundamentals of Nursing	5	3	2
Medical–Surgical Nursing I	7	4	3

Family Health Nursing	7	4	3
Psychiatric/Mental Health Nursing	5	3	2
Advanced Care Nursing	7	4	3
Acute Care	7	4	3
Chronic Care	7	4	3
Caring for the Community	7	4	3
Nursing Research I	3		
Historical Perspectives	3		
Pharmacology in Nursing	3		
Ethical and Legal Issues in Nursing	3		
Leadership and Trends in Nursing	3		
Transcultural Nursing or Holistic Nursing	3		
Transition to Professional Nursing Practice	3	1	2
TOTAL NURSING CREDITS	**73**		
SCHEDULE OF COURSES (FULL-TIME STUDENT}			
FIRST YEAR (FALL SEMESTER)			
	Course Credits	**Theory/Lecture**	**Clinical/Lab**
Fundamentals of Nursing I	5	3	2
Psychology I	3		
Anatomy and Physiology I	4	3	1
Nutrition	3		
English	3		
TOTAL CREDITS	**18**		
FIRST YEAR (SPRING SEMESTER)			
Medical–Surgical Nursing	5	3	2
Pharmacology	3		
Microbiology	3	2	1
Anatomy and Physiology II	3	2	1

Technology in Health Care	3		
TOTAL CREDITS	**17**		
SECOND YEAR (FALL SEMESTER)			
Psychiatric/Mental Health Nursing	5	3	2
Chemistry I	3	2	1
Sociology I	3		
Psychology II	3		
Historical Perspectives	3		
TOTAL CREDITS	**17**		
SECOND YEAR (SPRING SEMESTER)			
Maternal–Child Health Nursing	7	4	3
Organic Chemistry	3	2	1
Intermediate Algebra	3		
Elective (1)	3		
TOTAL CREDITS	**16**		
THIRD YEAR (FALL SEMESTER)			
Nursing Care of the Individual	7	4	3
Statistics for Social Sciences	3		
Transcultural Nursing or Holistic Nursing	3		
Elective (2)	3		
TOTAL CREDITS	**16**		
THIRD YEAR (SPRING SEMESTER)			
Family Centered Nursing	7	4	3
Nursing Research I	3		
Elective (3)	3		
TOTAL CREDITS	**13**		
FOURTH YEAR (FALL SEMESTER)			
Caring for the Community	7	4	3
Ethical and Legal Issues in Nursing	3		
Elective (4)	3		
TOTAL CREDITS	**13**		

FOURTH YEAR (SPRING SEMESTER)			
Critical Care Nursing	7	4	3
Transition to Professional Nursing Practice	3	1	2
Advanced Leadership in Nursing	3		
TOTAL CREDITS	**13**		
Total Credits for the Program	**126**		

Leveling the Constructs

Constructs: Program Outcomes	Level I	Level II	Level III	Level IV
Knowledge: Apply knowledge gained in the primary sciences courses to support nursing practice.	Demonstrate understanding of lifespan development.	Integrate pharmacological, biological, and pathophysiological aspects of health and illness in caring for families.	Implement pharmacological and pathophysiological concepts in managing health and illness in groups.	Synthesize the impact of environmental and biophysical factors on the care of client aggregates/communities.
Scientific research: Articulate identified problems in health care that lend themselves to clinical research.	Relate *Healthy People 2020* and current healthcare research to health promotion.	Identify current research findings that provide rationales for family-centered care.	Discuss current research findings that provide rationales for all levels of care.	Articulate identified problems in health care that lend themselves to clinical research. Develop research proposals.
Information management: Use information and communication technologies to enter, retrieve, and manipulate data for the delivery of health care.	Collect individual patient-specific healthcare information.	Analyze appropriate data to inform specific healthcare delivery.	Utilize appropriate data to plan care for all levels of clients.	Expand complex skills in retrieving and cross-checking healthcare data of aggregates/communities. Utilize findings to plan, implement, and evaluate care.

CHAPTER 4

Preparing for Classroom Teaching

OBJECTIVES

- Apply adult learning principles to the classroom setting.
- Develop course objectives utilizing Bloom's taxonomy.
- Utilize learning styles to develop classroom assignments.
- Design classroom activities to promote active and passive learning.

Teaching in the classroom or clinical setting for the first time will no doubt bring about several anxiety-provoking moments. Whether you are a new or an experienced faculty member, meeting your students for the first time can stir up conflicting emotions. Having an air of confidence and a relaxed attitude can be extremely beneficial when starting your first class. That aside, preparation is the key to success in the teaching environment.

As you begin your trip into academia, concentrate on the following. First, get a clear understanding of how college students learn. Next, understand some of the barriers that impede learning. Finally, be prepared to seek out strategies and techniques that promote learning. This may sound complex, but taking it one step at a time will help to make it meaningful.

Let us review how college students learn. Learning is a process of constructing meaningful representations (i.e., making sense of one's experiences). Learning involves a change in behavior and is often viewed as a process of becoming. Several different theories of learning are described in the literature; they can be made more understandable by grouping them into three main emphases—behavioral, cognitive, or constructivist.

The most popular **behaviorist theorists** are Albert Bandura, John B. Watson, B. F. Skinner, and Ivan Pavlov. Generally, behaviorist theories describe how learning occurs through observable behavior, how it can be reinforced by response, how it can be modified by modifying one's behavior, and how it is teacher centered. The onus lies on the teacher to model and reinforce behaviors that students are supposed to learn.

Cognitive theorists suggest that learning occurs as a function of the brain. Knowledge is created when information is received, processed, and stored in either long-term or short-term memory. This type of learning is student centered. Students are able to seek their own knowledge and build on previous knowledge. Cognitive theorists include Jean Piaget and Robert Gagne. Gagne's nine events of instruction identify internal processes that occur in the brain with each instructional event. As a practical example of these events, the teacher gains the attention of the student, describes the learning objectives, stimulates recall of prior learning, presents new content while guiding on what is to be learned, encourages psychomotor activities, gives feedback, assesses performance, and encourages retention and transfer. Concurrently, the brain is stimulated; the student reacts to the expectations; the information received stimulates short-term memory and there is recall of prior information; material to be remembered is received, stored, and processed; and periodic review leads to decreased loss of information from memory.

Constructivist theorists believe learning is actively constructed by the learner through interaction with the environment. This type of knowledge is marked by reflection and actions. This student-focused learning theory encourages the student to make sense of the world around her or him and determine what she or he views as important. The student's perspective of knowledge is gained through problem solving, reasoning, and critical thinking and does not have to be a reflection of the environment. How the student perceives the encounters is the most important factor. The most popular constructivist theorists are Jerome Bruner and Lev Vygotsky.

ADULT LEARNING PRINCIPLES

Undoubtedly you will be dealing with adult learners, so you will need to review the proper approach to teaching this group of students. The literature is replete with information regarding the ways in which adults learn. This is often referred to as *andragogy*, a term used to differentiate the adult process from how children learn (*pedagogy*). Brookfield (2012) describes four basic characteristics of the adult learner that incorporate most of the adult learning concepts reflected in the literature. First, adult learners come to the learning environment with multiple roles, responsibilities, and commitments. Second, adults typically learn throughout their lifetimes through negotiation and participation. Third, as they transition through different social and psychological experiences, adults redefine and rearrange the meanings of their life experiences. Finally, adults often have a level of anxiety and ambivalence in their approach to learning. Adults tend to learn more effectively at their own pace (Brookfield, 2012). They are self-directed, goal oriented, relevancy oriented, and practical, and require respect. It is important to incorporate adults' life situations into their current learning situations because past experiences tend to help them formulate their current interpretation of the world around them. Educators are aware that a safe environment is conducive to learning.

STRATEGIES FOR TEACHING THE ADULT LEARNER

First and foremost, adult learners need to feel that they are respected and that their previous life experiences can contribute meaningfully to the learning environment. Let them know that you are aware of the wealth of experiences they bring to the learning environment and that you will be expecting them to utilize prior experiences in solving problems. Create assignments that are less content centered, are experiential in nature, and allow for active versus passive participation; an example would be assigning students to practice interviewing each other in class rather than describing theoretically how interviews are carried out. Adult learners must feel that the information they are learning is meaningful and applicable to other areas of their lives.

TEACHING AND LEARNING STYLES

Students come to the classroom with prior knowledge and experiences that will impact how they fit into the educational environment and, ultimately, how they learn. Heredity, culture, and past experiences have tangible effects on how students learn. Additionally, students have expectations and challenges that can either enhance or impede their learning. These challenges may be attributed to, among other issues, cognitive, physical, social, or environmental causes. Cognitive reasons for difficulty in learning could include the inability to master content. Physical challenges may be related to hearing impairment, color blindness, dyslexia, or migraines. Social conditions could include the stressors of poverty or poor self-esteem. Finally, environmental barriers may include noise or poor lighting. Despite what the situation may be, the teacher has the responsibility to ensure that students are working toward meeting the course outcomes.

It is commonly believed that most teachers tend to teach the way they were taught; however, this may not be the best way to engage the students in their class. As a teacher you may want to begin by assessing the type of educator you are, determining your teaching style. There are many suggestions in the literature on how teachers can determine the type of educator they are. One suggestion is to complete the Colorado State University quiz (Colorado State University College of Business, n.d.). The result of this quiz identifies teachers as one of the following:

- *Demonstrators:* Those who coach and guide students by demonstrating what needs to be learned.
- *Facilitators:* Those who emphasize student-centered learning.
- *Delegators:* Those who place the emphasis of learning on the student. Students are expected to take responsibility to seek out knowledge.

Knowing what type of teacher you are will influence how you teach and manage your classroom.

Now that you know what type of educator you are, you can try to determine your learning style. Once again, there are several tools for measuring learning styles, but for simplicity and brevity we suggest completing the VARK learning style inventory (Vark-Learn, n.d.) on the VARK website. This inventory categorizes learners as follows:

- *Visual:* Those who learn best by seeing
- *Auditory:* Those who learn best by hearing
- *Read/write:* Those who learn best by writing and note taking
- *Tactile/kinesthetic:* Those who learn best through actually touching, doing, and moving

One of the first activities you should carry out when you meet a new class is to assess the students' learning styles to determine how congruent their styles are with your teaching style. Have each student complete the VARK learning style inventory. Knowing what their learning styles are will be of utmost importance in helping you focus on how best to teach them. The way you teach or your teaching style will also have a great impact on learning outcomes. You might have learned a great deal about the importance of learning styles in the past, but now you have ample opportunity to assess yours and your students' learning styles and to use this information to guide how you carry out classroom activities.

Although we suggest using the VARK learning inventory, we do not mean to suggest that one learning style is more valuable than the others. The concept is to have individuals recognize their personal learning strengths and weaknesses.

Note that the VARK assessment also can be used with students in the clinical setting; the results will guide instructors on how to appropriately assign students and evaluate their performances. Bearing in mind that students learn in different ways, the expected outcomes may vary. Faculty need to be flexible in adjusting clinical assignments to facilitate students' learning styles.

Several other learning styles tools are available in the literature. You should explore their content to make sure you are familiar with the material before self-administering or administering them to the students. Another commonly used inventory is the Kolb Learning Style Inventory, which can be obtained from Hay Resource Direct at www.haygroup.com/leadershipandtalentondemand/. The VARK assessment tool can be obtained from http://vark-learn.com/the-vark-questionnaire/. It is a quick and easy way to assess students' learning style while they are in the classroom. The test is done online and the results become available immediately.

Being aware of your own learning style will ensure that you incorporate other learning styles into your teaching and do not focus solely on what is most comfortable for you. Blevins (2014) reminds us that 80 percent of the general population are visual learners, meaning that they learn best when they are able to visualize the material being taught (e.g., on chalkboards, handouts, and overhead material). The remaining 20 percent of students benefit from other methods (e.g., verbal discussions, simulation, read/write). Recent studies suggest that a multimodal approach to teaching methods increases the likelihood of knowledge transfer in regard to changes in knowledge, healthcare practices, and subsequent patient outcomes (Curran, 2014).

In summary, faculty have a great responsibility to make sure that students are indeed learning in their classroom. What is even more important is that the teacher's teaching style is congruent with the student's learning style. Learning-style theorists generally believe that one's personality is related to how one learns. Learning styles are not fixed throughout life, but develop as people grow (Silver, Strong, & Perini, 1997). Other learning-style theorists agree that individuals practice a mixture of styles as they live and learn. Although it is impossible to identify each and every person's style of learning, if faculty use a variety of teaching strategies, everyone will benefit.

BLOOM'S TAXONOMY: DOMAINS OF LEARNING

When planning your lessons, it is important to include the expected outcomes regarding the course content. By clearly stating the objectives of the course you will be able to evaluate the course outcome. Being knowledgeable about the different domains of learning will be very beneficial when developing the course objectives. As a guide, we suggest you review Bloom's taxonomy. The following information is summarized from this website (http://academic.udayton.edu/health/syllabi/health/Unit01/lesson01b. htm), but there are several other interpretations of the taxonomy of learning.

Bloom's (Bloom et al., 2000) revised taxonomy is a well-known framework that describes three domains or categories of learning: cognitive, psychomotor, and affective. The **cognitive** domain is described as knowledge and the development of intellect. Within the cognitive domain are six main categories described in a hierarchical manner that reflects the direction in which knowledge is attained (see **Table 4-1**). The first step in the learning

TABLE 4-1 Cognitive Domain Categories	
Category	**Commonly Used Terms or Keywords**
Remembering: Can the student recall or remember the information?	Define, duplicate, list, memorize, recall, repeat, reproduce, state
Understanding: Can the student explain ideas or concepts?	Classify, describe, discuss, explain, identify, locate, paraphrase, recognize, report, select, translate
Applying: Can the student use the information in a new way?	Choose, demonstrate, dramatize, employ, illustrate, interpret, operate, schedule, sketch, solve, use, write
Analyzing: Can the student distinguish between the different parts?	Appraise, compare, contrast, criticize, differentiate, discriminate, distinguish, examine, experiment, question, test
Evaluating: Can the student justify a stand or decision?	Appraise, argue, defend, evaluate, judge, select, support, value
Creating: Can the student create a new product or point of view?	Assemble, construct, create, design, develop, formulate, write
Reproduced from Anderson, L. W., Krathwohl, D. R., Airasian, P. W., Cruikshank, K. A., Mayer, R. E., Pintrich, P. R.,. . . Wittrock, M. C. (2001). *A taxonomy for learning, teaching, and assessing: A revision of Bloom's taxonomy of educational objectives.* Upper Saddle River, NJ: Pearson.	

process is remembering, which involves the recall of data (repeats, lists, recalls, recognizes), followed by understanding the data (explains, gives examples, translates, paraphrases). The next step, applying, refers to the student's ability to do something (computes, modifies, uses constructs), followed by analyzing the material into component parts (appraises, compares, contrasts, criticizes, differentiates). Students distinguish between facts and inferences. Next, in evaluating (appraises, argues, defends, judges, selects), students create a new meaning. Finally, during the process of creating (assembles, constructs, creates, designs, develops), judgments about the value of ideas or material are made. The overall objective of any curriculum is to ensure that knowledge is acquired to varying degrees. Formative and summative examinations are developed to measure to what degree knowledge formation takes place.

The **affective** domain of learning deals with how one handles things emotionally. There are five main categories in this domain, which are accompanied by keywords that can be used as you integrate this domain into the curriculum.

The first category deals with how one receives information and the level of attention and awareness (acknowledges, asks, listens). The second category deals with responsiveness or active participation (assists, discusses, presents, tells). Valuing, the third category, ranges from simple acceptance to complex commitment (demonstrates, differentiates, justifies, respects). The fourth category, prioritization, accepts professional ethical standards (compares, relates, synthesizes). Finally, the fifth category, characterization or the internalizing of values, demonstrates behaviors that are consistent, pervasive, and predictable (discriminates, displays, influences, performs). In this domain, students will demonstrate a change in behavior or feeling related to new knowledge. Empathy is emphasized.

The **psychomotor** domain deals with the accomplishment of motor skills through physical movement. There are seven major categories that involve speed, precision, and practice:

- *Perception:* The ability to use sensory cues to guide motor activities (chooses, describes, distinguishes, selects)
- *Set:* Demonstrating readiness to act mentally, physically, or emotionally (moves, begins, reacts, volunteers)
- *Guided response:* Achieving by practice or trial and error (copies, traces, follows, reproduces)
- *Mechanism:* Intermediate stage of learning where there is some level of confidence in skill performance (assembles, calibrates, organizes)
- *Complex overt response:* Proficiency in completing skills with a minimum of energy; able to perform without hesitation (assembles, builds, manipulates, fixes)
- *Adaptation:* Well-developed skills with the ability to modify certain areas (adapts, alters, reorganizes, rearranges)
- *Origination:* Demonstrating creativity based on highly developed skills (arranges, builds, creates, designs)

Students demonstrate competency in this domain by carrying out skills with speed, precision, and confidence.

DIVERSITY IN THE CLASSROOM

The word *diversity* conjures up thoughts about differences in sex, age, race, ethnicity, culture, and outward physical appearance. In the classroom, these are more or less the obvious or visible diverse characteristics that are observable at first glance. The classroom, however, is replete with a variety of unobservable or hidden student characteristics that may not be easily identified by the teacher or students. These are referred to broadly as *hidden diversities* and include such characteristics as lifestyle preferences, language/speech differentiation, national origin, learning disabilities, time orientation, and the various learning styles mentioned previously. Diversity of thoughts and diversity of previous experiences are now being given a great deal of attention in the literature. Embracing these two concepts enriches the classroom experience for all involved and also creates an inclusive atmosphere.

The teacher must be committed to fostering an inclusive climate that respects all groups, no matter what their race, color, ethnicity, age, and other characteristics. This does not always occur, and it is not inconceivable that a faculty member may be well intentioned yet still be perceived as being biased (Savini, 2010). Becoming aware of your own unconscious biases is an important step in diminishing the appearance of being insensitive to your students. One suggestion is for new faculty to consider taking the Four-Category Race IAT assessment (Project Implicit, 2012).

Being aware of your unconscious biases will allow you to compensate by using appropriate language, applying decision-making and teaching strategies that cannot be perceived as offensive to any group, and respecting behaviors that may reflect students' personal orientation. Employing open, honest communication strategies and respect for all students is one clear way faculty can decrease the impact of bias in the classroom.

One other area that you should be aware of is gender bias in written texts. Often male nurses' contributions to the profession are subtly overlooked. The literature is replete with information regarding gender bias, discrimination, and inequality in the nursing profession. Suggested readings are Ross (2008) and Anthony (2004).

PASSIVE AND ACTIVE LEARNING

Passive and active teaching strategies are opposite methods of teaching. In the passive or traditional way of teaching/learning, students are provided with the material to be learned in a written or didactic format, such as texts, handouts, and other educational material. Teaching takes place mainly in the classroom or via the web. The power in the teaching/learning environment lies with the teacher. In other words, the experience is more teacher focused. Students' participation is minimal—they are expected to pay attention to learning the material as presented.

The active teaching/learning environment is one of interaction, participation, and engagement. Students are challenged to use high levels of critical thinking and decision making. The learning is student focused, and students are expected to familiarize themselves with the material and have input in discussing it during class. It is believed that this type of learning stimulates the higher cognitive processes. There are, however, pros and cons to both ways of teaching/learning.

Despite what many believe, research shows that passive learning is the preferred learning method for many students because it tends to be less anxiety provoking, allowing students to feel more secure. Having been given the information beforehand, students come prepared to learn in a controlled environment. This method of teaching is also advantageous for some teachers, especially new faculty who are able to provide a vast amount of information in a limited period of time in a comfortable environment. This way of teaching allows for a concrete, organized way of delivering information.

There are, however, some noted disadvantages to this traditional way of teaching/learning. Despite students' appreciation of having the material provided to them ahead of time, some report feeling there is little time during class for clarification of the material or for discussions and questions. Students may also be reluctant to ask questions in class, thereby leading to false assumptions by faculty that the students have a full grasp of the material. Faculty, for their part, may appear to be tedious and boring to the students as they spend time repeating material that some students have previously reviewed (VickyRN, 2009).

In active learning, students are involved at all levels of the learning process through feedback, operations, and input. Students demonstrate initiative in gathering, discussing, and demonstrating understanding of the material; they verbally interact with each other and the teacher, so their voices are heard and their contributions to the discourse are acknowledged. They have the opportunity to bring previous experiences into the discussion, making the class a more interactive and interesting environment. Teachers have a great opportunity to direct the conversation as they stimulate students' critical-thinking and decision-making skills. This method of teaching/learning can capture a variety of learning styles such as visual, verbal, auditory, kinesthetic, and interpersonal. During these interactions, the teacher has a better opportunity to assess how students are learning.

There are, however, some disadvantages to the active way of teaching/learning. This type of learning may be stressful to some students who have been steeped in the traditional way of learning. Classroom participation may bring about unnecessary distress for some. New faculty, who may be just learning the material to be covered, may find this style of teaching more challenging than do experienced faculty who have a vast knowledge of the material. As a result, new faculty will need to expend a vast amount of time and energy to learn the material, organize active learning experiences, and direct the classroom activities. In the initial phases of introducing active learning strategies, students may be somewhat uncomfortable in adapting to the format; as a result, student evaluation of faculty may reflect this maladaptation.

Experts are now leaning toward the active way of learning as the preferred modality, but studies show that traditional didactic and passive strategies are still perceived as being valuable to some students. Nevertheless, we must remember that there are advantages and disadvantages to both types of teaching/learning, as well as other compounding factors that will impact how students learn. The classroom represents diverse student demographics, which must be taken into consideration when planning the curriculum. A mixture of active and passive strategies is recommended, as is a degree of flexibility on the part of the faculty. Using the adult learning principles as a guide in developing the curriculum will allow faculty to take into consideration students' previous experiences, their attitudes toward learning, and their personality types (VickyRN, 2009).

PREPARING TO LECTURE

The goal of most teachers is to provide information in a format that will ensure student learning. Contrary to some popular opinions, students rate the lecture as a very acceptable way to learn. Lecturing is regarded as a passive way of learning that is teacher focused. Nevertheless, it has proved to be a convenient traditional teaching strategy that is overwhelmingly employed in many schools and colleges, especially among faculty new to academia or when dealing with new material, as well as when it is necessary to provide a large amount of material in a short period of time. Never underestimate the power and effectiveness of the lecture.

An effective lecture must be well prepared and delivered. It is estimated that it takes approximately eight hours to prepare a one-hour lecture. It may take even longer when dealing with new and unfamiliar material. Preparing a lecture calls for researching the content, organizing the material into a cohesive whole, preparing audiovisuals, creating student handouts and other resources, ensuring the presence and functionality of audiovisual equipment, and arranging the classroom for maximum comfort and learning. It is not sufficient for the teacher to read only from the assigned text, because this may become quite boring for the listeners. Instead, the teacher must gather relevant information on the topic from a variety of sources and spend time comparing and contrasting. Point out to students that material in most assigned texts may have taken several years to develop, so information may have changed or may need to be updated.

Now you are prepared and ready to teach. Provide the students with a syllabus with clear objectives and a detailed reading outline. Most schools require that course syllabi are prepared long before the start of the semester. The syllabi will contain the course schedule, reading assignments, and some course policies. In many cases this information is provided to the student before the start of class. Syllabi may be posted on standard course management platforms such as MOODLE, Blackboard, or WebCT. If these platforms are not used at your school, then it is quite appropriate to email each student the syllabus or have students pick up a hard copy from your office prior to the start of class. This will make it easier for you to go over the information with them on the first day of class. Students will also have the opportunity to review the syllabus and print a copy to bring with them to the classroom. Often they will secure their syllabus prior to the first day of classes, review the list of required and recommended reading, and buy their text(s), and they often will have questions or need clarification. The general structure and layout of a syllabus is described in Chapter 3.

You are now challenged to engage the students and keep them focused on the material being presented. Before starting, you will need to develop a positive rapport with the students using icebreakers or other strategies that will be discussed later in this chapter. Reassure the students that the learning environment is a safe place where all are respected and all voices will be heard. Bearing in mind how adults learn, keep the material relevant, practical, and evidence based, allowing time for clarification and discussions.

Suggestions for Prior to the Start of Class

Preparing your classroom to receive your students is of utmost importance. These efforts convey to the students that they are expected and are welcomed. Starting off on a positive note will result in a more positive experience for all. This positive attitude will present to the students a welcoming environment. Here are some hints that you may find helpful:

1. Arrange desks and chairs in a semicircle where everyone is able to have a clear view of everyone else and communication can be direct.
2. Have students give brief introductions (name, employment, reason for taking the class).
3. Ask students if they have questions or need clarification.
4. Reaffirm that everyone has the assigned reading material.
5. Suggest students write any unanswered questions on a piece of paper that you will collect at the end of class and clarify at the start of the next class.

During Class: Primacy/Recency

Psychologists believe the order in which material is presented will impact the quality and quantity of what is remembered. Material presented earlier is better remembered than material presented later on. This effect is known as *primacy*. Conversely, students tend to be able to recall the most recent information taught (*recency*). Therefore, the material presented somewhere in the middle of the lecture tends to be least remembered. The suggestion for the teacher, therefore, is to organize material so that the most important concepts of the lecture are presented either early on or toward the end. An effective lecture should be delivered as follows: *Prime time 1* occurs during the first part of the class, followed by a period of *down time* where material that is least critical is taught, and then the lecture ends with *prime time 2*. The middle or down-time period can be used for discussion, viewing movies, and group work.

The following is an example of implementing the primacy/recency strategy for a four-hour pharmacology lecture:

- *Prime time 1:* The first two hours are used to identify the physiologic responses of specific drugs on the central nervous system, and compare and contrast the mechanisms of action of cholinergic agonists.
- *Down time:* Watch a 30-minute video on patients' behavior while taking anticholinergics, followed by discussion, questions, and answers.
- *Prime time 2:* Provide a PowerPoint presentation of a list of anticholinergics and their indications, side effects, and nursing implications. This is followed by discussions.

TEACHING STRATEGIES THAT PROMOTE PASSIVE LEARNING

The transfer of information from the teacher's thinking to the student involves passive student participation. No particular effort is made to bring the information down to the student's level of comprehension (Tedesco-Schneck, 2013). Examples of assignments that lead to passive learning include

- Podium lectures
- Videos and movies
- PowerPoint slides
- Chalkboard assignments

TEACHING STRATEGIES THAT PROMOTE ACTIVE LEARNING

In the active classroom, the teacher provides students with opportunities to participate and learn at the same time. The literature provides hundreds of strategies that promote active learning (Teaching Community, n.d.). You may want to become familiar with a variety of strategies that are applicable to your classroom and to use different ones depending on what is being taught and the content to be learned. The following are some strategies that are commonly used in the nursing classroom along with examples on how to use them:

- Icebreakers are typically used in the initial class meeting with the goal of creating a positive, welcoming environment; relaxing participants; and setting the tone for future classes. The following are some examples of icebreakers:
  - Tell the class something funny about yourself and then go around the room asking each student to do the same.
  - Go around the room, have each student call out his or her name, and then ask everyone to list as many names as they can remember.
  - Start a sentence such as "I want to be a nurse because. . ." and have each student complete it.
  - Have each student guess the teacher's birthday and write it on a piece of paper. Collect the papers and hand out a token prize to the person who came closest.
- Case studies are commonly used to cover material that students have previously experienced either in the classroom or in the clinical setting. They are often based on real-life scenarios. The goal of case studies is to have students develop their skills in analytic reasoning and reflective judgment. Teachers get the chance to evaluate their students' critical thinking and evaluate student learning. Case studies may be long passages or short, two-line sentences that are designed so that students are prompted to ask questions as the case unfolds. Often there are unanswered questions that call for further research. The most interesting cases are those that are drawn from real-life experiences; therefore, you should design cases that students are more likely to see or experience in the clinical setting.
- Student presentations have two main purposes. First, they give students the opportunity to carry out work outside of the classroom and bring the information back to share with the class. Second, they help to develop students' organizational and preparatory skills. Students demonstrate their ability to communicate publicly. The teacher gets to evaluate the student's knowledge, ability, and critical thinking and give real-time feedback in a positive manner. The teacher's responsibility is to give clear written directions regarding the overall expectations for the presentation. Whenever possible, a grading rubric should be given to the students along with the presentation assignment. Graded presentations tend to be better prepared than ungraded ones.
- Simulation in the classroom and laboratory settings has become quite popular over the past decade. Simulation refers to the replication of an experience

commonly found in a clinical setting, using a manikin or other resource. You can use simulation to demonstrate skills and experiences that may be missed in the clinical setting. It provides a safe environment for students to practice prior to going into the clinical site. Active learners find simulation to be an effective tool that encourages interaction, allows for individually paced learning, and provides an opportunity for students to practice on their own. There are three levels of simulations: low, medium, and high fidelity. The most cost-effective simulations are the static or low-fidelity ones, which are commonly used in classroom labs to practice procedural skills. Medium-fidelity skills can also be used for procedural skills but are more interactive. High-fidelity simulators are expensive but provide full-scale, computer-integrated, and physiologically responsive manikins. Students' experiences with these simulators are designed to be similar to clinical experiences in clinical sites.

- Independent study assignments provide opportunities for active learners to think critically, explore options, be flexible, collaborate outside of the classroom, and be creative in their learning. When giving independent study assignments, the teacher must be careful to allow students to be flexible in thoughts and actions. If the assignment is to be graded, students should be given a rubric along with the assignment to guide their work.
- Concept maps consist of illustrations that show the relationships among concepts. They are designed to help students develop logical thinking as they explore the linkages between ideas, resulting in an understanding of the big picture. Concept maps are visual representations of the relationships between ideas or concepts where each word or idea connects to another and links back to the original word or idea. The pictorial diagram shows the link between concepts. As a learning tool, concept maps allow for critical thinking and rationalization. Each concept in the map is represented by a figure such as a square, triangle, or circle; the figures are joined by lines with labeled arrows demonstrating the direction in which the link is occurring. Recently, the concept map has been replacing the traditional nursing care plans and is viewed as a strategy that provides the opportunity for students to increase their critical-thinking and decision-making skills. As a teaching tool, the concept map allows students to explore ideas, build a body of knowledge around a particular subject, explore relationships, expand on prior knowledge, and then present a view of the entire content.
- Flipping the classroom is a student-centered method of teaching that has gained popularity over the past decade; however, it has been in existence for decades, especially in graduate studies. By flipping the classroom, reversed teaching strategies can lead to increased learning, while bringing about new and more exciting learning outcomes. In the flipped model of classes, students are held accountable for accessing course content outside of the classroom. Faculty may

design content or direct students to appropriate content that must be covered prior to coming to class. Students have the opportunity to acquire the information by reviewing faculty-prepared audiovisuals, reading the text, exploring the web, or similar sources. In other words, students can choose from a variety of sources and determine which is most conducive to the way they learn. During the class, students have the opportunity to spend individual time working with professors on what they have learned so far. In the classroom, teachers can use strategies such as case studies, narrative pedagogy, questions and answers, or discussion to cover the material. This type of classroom gives students the opportunity to express themselves in less formal ways and heightens peer-to-peer and teacher interactions.

- In team-based learning, students are assigned to teams or groups to discuss and explore the material either in class or on their own time. This method is sometimes controversial, especially when group members are unable to come to consensus regarding the content or process. There are many variations in how team-based learning can be effective. Recently, Brame (2014) discussed an approach to team-based test taking. A group of five to seven students take tests individually and then take the test as a group. Following the group testing there is intense discussion and negotiation on how the students arrived at the correct answers (Brame, 2014). This method of learning has the added benefit of increased student-to-student and student-to-faculty interactions.

CASE STUDY

You are newly hired pediatric faculty for the Department of Nursing at a local university. You are assigned to teach the pediatric course to level-three nursing students. The syllabus for this course needs to be revised to reflect the IOM report and *The Future of Nursing*.

1. Develop the course objectives.
2. Identify the teaching strategies you will use throughout the classroom component of this course to address the learning needs of a diverse population of students.
3. Plan student assignments to measure course objectives.

REFERENCES

Anderson, L. W., Krathwohl, D. R., Airasian, P. W., Cruikshank, K. A., Mayer, R. E., Pintrich, P. R., . . . Wittrock, M. C. (2000). *Taxonomy for learning, teaching, and assessing: A revision of Bloom's taxonomy of educational objectives* (1st ed.). New York, NY: Longman.

Anthony, A. S. (2004). Gender bias and discrimination in nursing education. Can we change it? *Nurse Educator, 29*, 121–125.

Blevins, S. (2014). Understanding learning styles. *MedSurg Nursing, 23*(1), 59–60.

Brame, C. (2014). Team-based learning: What is it? Retrieved from http://cft.vanderbilt.edu/guides-sub-pages/team-based-learning

Brookfield, S. D. (2012). *Teaching for critical thinking: Tools and techniques to help student question their assumptions.* San Francisco, CA: Jossey Bass Higher Education.

Colorado State University College of Business. (n.d.). What is your teaching style? Retrieved from http://www.biz.colostate.edu/mti/tips/pages/WhatisYourTeachingStyle.aspx

Curran, M. K. (2014). Examination of the teaching styles of nursing professional development specialists, part I: Best practices in adult learning theory, curriculum development, and knowledge transfer. *Journal of Continuing Education in Nursing, 45*(5), 233–240. doi:10.3928/00220124-20140417-04

Project Implicit. (2012). Featured task: Four-Category Race IAT. Retrieved from https://implicit.harvard.edu/implicit/user/featuredtasks/race4/featuredtask.html

Ross, H. (2008). Proven strategies for addressing unconscious bias in the workplace. *Diversity Best Practices, 2*(5).

Savini, C. (2010). Bias among the well-intentioned: How it can affect the hiring process. *Independent School, 69*(2). Retrieved from http://www.nais.org/Magazines-Newsletters/ISMagazine/Pages/Bias-Among-the-Well-Intentioned.aspx

Silver, H. F., Strong, R. W., & Perini, M. J. (1997). Integrating learning styles and multiple intelligences. *Educational Leadership, 55*(1), 22–27.

Teaching Community. (n.d.). 40 active learning strategies for active students. Retrieved from http://teaching.monster.com/benefits/articles/8414-40-active-learning-strategies-for-active-students-?page=2

Tedesco-Schneck, M. (2013). Active learning as a path to critical thinking: Are competencies a roadblock? *Nurse Education in Practice, 13*(1), 58–60. doi:10.1016/j.nepr.2012.07.007

VARK Learn Limited. (n.d.). The VARK questionnaire: How do I learn best? Retrieved from http://www.vark-learn.com/the-vark-questionnaire

VickyRN. (2009, April 2). From teaching to learning: The advantages of passive vs. active learning strategies. Retrieved from http://allnurses.com/nursing-educators-faculty/teaching-learning-advantages-382190.html

CHAPTER 5

Classroom Environment

OBJECTIVES

- Create a plan to manage the classroom setting and facilitate student–faculty relationships given the physical environment, class size, and student diversity.
- Identify signs of incivility in the classroom.
- Explain faculty and student rights and responsibilities in the classroom.

This chapter describes all facets of the educational environment that facilitate learning. The educator has the responsibility to develop and implement a variety of teaching strategies and create a learning environment that is conducive to learning, is safe and nonjudgmental, and affords students the opportunity to develop mentally as well as socially.

THE CLASSROOM ENVIRONMENT

Traditionally the classroom environment is regarded as the physical setting, combined with the psychological, social, and instructional experiences related to teacher–student characteristics and behaviors. The classroom environment plays as important a part in the teaching/learning experience as the content being learned. The environment consists of teachers, students, relationships, behaviors, abilities, competencies, and individuals. When any part of the environment is out of synch, there can be a big impact on learning outcomes. As a new instructor, it is advisable to be cognizant of all aspects of the environment to have positive academic outcomes.

Recent research has explored the psychosocial impact of student–teacher relationships and student–student relationships on educational outcomes. Educators have adjusted classroom environments and teaching modalities over time to accommodate what evidence has shown to be effective.

THE PHYSICAL ENVIRONMENT

Let us start with the physical environment, which can influence behavioral and academic outcomes. You may have little control over the physical location in which you teach, but there are still a few suggestions that will help you enhance students' comfort and maximize learning. The classroom should be arranged so that every student has a clear view of and access to the teacher. The physical configuration of the furniture should match the type of interaction planned for the day. It sometimes may be necessary to arrange the classroom in a circle or semicircle. The lighting should be adequate and all students should be able to see what is being projected or written on the board. Always check your classroom before the students arrive to ensure that all equipment is functioning appropriately. It can be very disheartening if your audiovisual equipment fails just as you are about to begin teaching. The same can be said of online teaching. Make sure your technology is fully functioning before starting your chat sessions. Resources such as projector equipment, smartboards, desks and chairs, and computers must be fully functional. Educators are frequently engaged in using technology such as iPads, tablet PCs, and a variety of social media in the classroom to enhance teaching and encourage student learning.

Class size is usually determined by the scope of the curriculum. It is not unusual for faculty to be assigned upward of 50 students in a class; however, studies suggest that a class size of 30 or less is most conducive to learning. Smaller class sizes allow students to be less stressed, more cooperative, more attentive, and on task with assignments. Larger class sizes, by comparison, tend to have students who are more stressed, less cooperative, more distracted, more inattentive, and more anxious, and in some cases they have poorer educational outcomes. The larger the class, the more preparation you may have to do. If you are carrying out a very interactive class, you may find that the discussions and the desire of everyone to be heard may result in high levels of confusion that may even lead to disruption. Dividing the class into smaller groups and allowing one group to speak at a time may result in fewer interruptions.

Class composition may also significantly impact your class. It should not be surprising if in the traditional nursing classroom you come across more female than male students. The current male-to-female ratio in nursing is approximately 1:10. This should not make much difference in how and what you teach; however, the interactions may differ from those in non-nursing classrooms. You may also have a variety of learners in terms of age and learning speed. Older adults often take longer to digest what is being asked; therefore, special considerations need to be made for them. There will no doubt be a diverse group of students in the classroom. Diversity may be found in terms of age, sex, race, sexual orientation, ideas, learning styles, and intelligence. Although at first the level of diversity may be challenging, soon you will begin to see how interesting the dialogue will become.

CLASSROOM MANAGEMENT

To have an effective classroom, you must start out by managing it in the way you would like it to be for the entire semester. A classroom that is effectively run will afford students the social support they need and the mutual respect that all deserve. As a teacher you need to set boundaries. This is not only a good habit, but also a part of growth and development. By setting limits and boundaries you help the students organize their lives in a meaningful way. They learn to plan their studies as well as meet deadlines, which as you know is a part of everyday life.

Start by having clear goals and expectations for the class. These can be written in the syllabus, verbally stated on the first day of class, or given in a **written contract**. Having a written contract between the teacher and the students is one way to hold everyone accountable to classroom expectations. The contract can outline the expectations for behaviors to be adhered to and the consequences of not adhering to those behaviors. Students must be consistently held accountable. Topics that can be included in a contract can be related to lateness, absenteeism, class participation, and grading. If students are not permitted to enter your class after a certain start time, then you must stick to that rule. If a grade is provided for class participation and a student does not participate, then she or he should not receive that grade point.

In the same manner in which you hold your students accountable, you should also hold yourself accountable. Make it a habit to be prompt, organized, engaging, and interesting to the students.

DIVERSITY IN THE CLASSROOM

Dealing with a diverse student population brings its own challenges. Following are some insights and suggestions on how teachers can address students of diverse ages, sexes, sexual orientations, races, and religions.

Approach the class with an open mind free of preconceived ideas and biases. Always anticipate issues surrounding sexuality, religion, and other values. One false assumption some teachers make is that all minority students of a certain race have a collective identity (Trustees of Indiana University, 2010). This could not be further from the truth. Therefore, do not ignore students' individuality by singling out one student to speak on behalf of a specific group or to receive any special attention or favors. Monitor students' commentaries to defuse any personal attacks. Finally, in making or giving assignments, be aware of people's values and beliefs in regard to cultural expectations and religious affiliations; for example, do not assign a male Muslim student to care for a Jewish woman in labor because this may be prohibited.

Whether in the classroom or online, remain aware of undertones during discussions. If you notice there is a tendency for some students to make personal attacks on another's race, religion, sexual orientation, or the like, you must interject immediately, pointing out that such behavior is unacceptable.

When forming groups, take advantage of the rich cultural diversity in the classroom by assigning students to groups of different ages, sexes, ethnicities, religions, cultures, and abilities. This will result in deeper discussions and understandings among students.

Be fair and unbiased in your management of the classroom. Students, especially those who are failing, often accuse the teacher of being unfair and in some cases biased against them. Having such feelings can negatively impact the way students learn.

Spending an appropriate amount of time at the beginning of the semester explaining and discussing the classroom expectations will significantly decrease the amount of time you will have to spend later in the semester dealing with issues related to classroom conduct. When all students know the rules, it is less likely the teacher will be seen as being unfair.

FACULTY–STUDENT RELATIONSHIPS

The basis of positive student–faculty relationships is open communication. Studies by Arielli and colleagues (2012) and Dapremont (2014) demonstrate the importance of open communication between faculty and students so that optimal learning can occur. The relationship that develops between students and faculty creates the psychological environment. Positive relationships between faculty and students result in increased class participation. Students view teachers as role models. Teachers who are seen as positive, caring, respectful, committed, and supportive in all aspects of the student's learning tend to have students who are motivated and engaged. The students view the classroom as being socially supportive. For students to feel confident in their abilities and to be engaged in using all the resources and strategies presented by the teacher, there must be a feeling of mutual respect. The more time spent encouraging the student, the more likely the student will focus on completing assignments and participating in classwork.

Encourage meaningful dialogue with students so they feel their opinions matter; by doing so you will find that you spend less time responding to individual questions. Patrick, Ryan, and Kaplan (2007) report that students who receive frequent encouragement and emotional support from their teachers are more likely to focus on completing their tasks.

Finally, remember to keep a close watch on your nonverbal communication in the classroom. Nonverbal communication can be demonstrated by physical posture, clothing, eye contact, facial expressions, tone of voice, and the distance held between students and teachers. Several of these ways of communicating can be threatening to students. For example, according to De Freitas Castro Carrari de Amorim and Da Silva (2014), if you are pacing at the front of the classroom with your "chin up and hands crossed behind your back, you are displaying superiority," (p. 195) which could be intimidating to a group of new nursing students.

Strategies for Facilitating Student Involvement in the Classroom

Students are expected to leave the classroom having gained knowledge, skills, and attitudes as they strive to meet educational outcomes. The level of student involvement and participation in the classroom is not a given; therefore, it is important for teacher and student to work together to create and nurture a positive relationship. Whether you are teaching in a lecture or discussion format, the goal should be to elicit student participation. You cannot expect to have all students participate at the same level in each session because interest often waxes and wanes. Nevertheless, there should be opportunities for all students to participate at some level.

As the teacher, your first goal is to create a *safe environment* where everyone feels safe to express their views. By doing so you will be able to assess the level of comprehension or misunderstanding that is taking place in your classroom. Suggested strategies are to assess the class environment, plan activities that will facilitate involvement, create an environment that will maximize student involvement, and perform ongoing evaluation of the level of student involvement.

As you **assess** students for their level of participation, you should bear in mind that not all students can be spontaneous in their reactions; some may need more time to reflect on questions before coming up with answers. Other students, in contrast, may be spontaneous and reactive. Therefore you should initially take some time to assess the makeup of the classroom environment and plan accordingly. You will no doubt have students who are verbal—some may even try to manipulate the classroom; you will also have quiet students who are uncomfortable speaking publicly, and in the extreme, some who may feel alienated or marginalized. Try to engage each student, giving all students the support and reassurance they need to express themselves. The use of technology in the classroom has been shown to facilitate student involvement in the learning process. Chapter 12 is dedicated to describing several technological strategies that can enhance student engagement.

Plan to present the content in a variety of formats throughout the semester. You may want to present mini-lectures during a discussion course or discussions during a lecture course. Short, one-paragraph written assignments during class that are then discussed at the end of the class can also help to break up the monotony and keep students engaged. Group assignments have controversial support but do encourage intergroup communication and collaboration. Students have become extremely technologically savvy and seem to thrive in a technology-friendly environment. Having students access the web during class to search for the most current information on the topic being presented can also bring about heightened levels of excitement and involvement.

Practical strategies include getting to know all students and addressing them by their names as often as possible. This will give the students a feeling of belonging and at the same time decrease their anxiety. They may also feel a desire to participate when they are being personally acknowledged. Have students introduce themselves to each other and encourage them to get to know each other outside of class. The more students are familiar with each other, the less intimidated they will feel about participating in the classroom.

Questions and answers form the basis for student engagement. The teacher's verbal and nonverbal approach to questions and answers will help determine students' level of anxiety. When you ask a question, make sure everyone feels like it is being asked of them and not to any particular person or persons in the room. Make eye contact with all students. Do not always choose the first person who raises a hand, especially if that person appears to want to manipulate the classroom. Give everyone a chance to think through the question and formulate an answer. Often a quiet student may be thinking about the answer and need more time to come up with it. Give students enough time to think through the question and encourage them to take a shot at it. Refrain from answering your own question too quickly before giving adequate time for a response. This may discourage students from formulating their own answers. It is important to articulate your question well, rephrasing if necessary, and to listen carefully to what the student has to say before responding. If necessary, repeat the question and the answer to the class, asking if everyone agrees or if someone else has something else to add to the response.

Strategies for classroom management include the following:

- Have students openly introduce themselves on the first day of class.
- Get to know all students and address them by name as soon as possible.
- Be aware of your verbal and nonverbal cues.
- Encourage all students to participate by calling on different students at different times.
- Allow adequate time for students to respond to your questions.
- Acknowledge everyone's opinion.

NURSING CODE OF ETHICS

A very important text for all nurses to be familiar with is the *Guide to the Code of Ethics for Nurses*, edited by Marsha D. M. Fowler (2008) and published by the American Nurses Association. This text outlines nine codes for practicing nurses in all disciplines along with interpretative statements and applications. These codes emphasize the ethical practice of nurses, the nurse's commitment to protect the health and safety of the patient, the nurse's accountability to individual practice, the nurse's responsibility for maintaining competency and advancing the profession, and the nurse's responsibility to articulate values, maintain the integrity of the profession, and shape social policy. These codes are intended for the practicing nurse; however, nursing students also need to be aware of these codes early in their career, and it is the responsibility of faculty to pass these on.

MANAGING THE DISRUPTIVE/UNCIVIL STUDENT

Incivility in the classroom involves behavior that is unprofessional and often disruptive. Such behaviors compromise the learning environment as well as obstruct safe, quality client care. Disruptive behaviors may be encountered from student to student, student to faculty, faculty to student, or faculty to faculty. Most schools have policies and student codes of conduct that outline expectations for students in the classroom. The list of unacceptable behaviors includes, but is not limited to, physical threats, obscenities, verbal abuse of the teacher, outbursts or any other behavior that disrupts the teaching/learning environment, and stalking.

What causes a student to display uncivil, disruptive behavior in the classroom or clinical setting? Unruly behavior in the classroom or clinical setting can often be linked to deeper problems than meet the eye. Students often are tense due to heightened competition, personal stress factors, competing responsibilities, and difficulty with adjustment. They may lash out at each other as well as faculty. Some can be quite subtle with their hostility, whereas others cannot contain themselves. Occasionally you may come across students who consistently demonstrate disruptive behavior in the classroom and clinical sites.

Incivility in the classroom can take many forms (see **Box 5-1**), ranging from passive–aggressive behavior, inattentiveness, and talking among themselves to intimidating behavior. In the extreme you may encounter bullying, rudeness, disrespect, verbal outbursts, and threats or even physical attacks. Such behaviors are usually at odds with ethical practice and can place patients and colleagues at high risk for injury and

---

Box 5-1 Signs of Incivility in the Classroom

- Inattentiveness
- Passive–aggressive behavior
- Talking among themselves
- Abusiveness
- Bullying
- Verbal outbursts
- Threats
- Disrespect
- Physical attacks

harm. Should you be faced with such a situation, it is imperative that you intervene immediately, remain calm so as not to cause the situation to escalate, remove the student from the environment if necessary, and refer the student to the correct campus support division. Depending on how serious the incident is, you may request a private meeting with the student after class. "An important step in de-escalating conflicts and curtailing incivilities is listening to students to understand their perceptions and feelings" (Altmiller, 2012, p. 1). This may improve the student–professor relationship by forming a foundation based on trust and interest in the student's well-being.

When questioned, students often will address their academic performance as the root cause of their behavior rather than the underlying social issues. Students should be referred to the appropriate office for counseling and other resources such as anger management, student assistance, and psychological counseling. In most schools these services are available through the Office of Special Services (OSS). Students who consistently display disruptive behaviors should be reported to the school and be monitored for improvement in behavior once they have received the appropriate intervention. If the student was dismissed from the classroom, he or she must present a letter of clearance from the OSS before being allowed back into the classroom.

Often faculty consider incivility as solely a student behavior, but students often also describe incivility as coming from the teacher. Be aware that students can feel they have been treated uncivilly when a teacher is unprepared for class, is late, is disruptive, speaks in an aggressive tone, is unavailable after classes, does not appreciate students' efforts, is unreasonable, is demeaning, or belittles students (Clark & Springer, 2010). Do not respond to emails or phone calls inappropriately, or demonstrate inappropriate body language while teaching.

You may not be able to identify which student will demonstrate a particular behavior (see **Table 5-1**), but be prepared to react in an appropriate way. Snyder (2010) suggests that all teachers keep safety in mind first and foremost. Respond by calmly asking the explosive student to calm down and remain seated. If the behavior persists, then security should be called in. In the case of a passive–aggressive or antisocial student, you should meet with the student privately and point out the behavior. Discuss the root cause and how you can best work with that student. Always refer to the school's policy on disruptive behaviors.

Faculty-to-faculty incivility is not unheard of, and if this behavior is observed by students it can have a negative effect on the learning environment.

Additionally, students have reported faculty unfairness, rigidity, insistence on conformity, and overt discrimination as behaviors contributing to academic incivility. Consequences of this behavior include disrupted student–faculty relationships, problematic learning environments, and increased stress levels among students and faculty (Clark & Springer, 2010).

TABLE 5-1 Characteristics of Disruptive Students	
Characteristic	**Behaviors**
Explosive	Bullying, volatile, threatening
Antisocial	Cheats, steals, forges, exploits others
Passive–aggressive	Chronically late, sleeps in class, procrastinates
Narcissistic	Arrogant, self-centered, entitled, devalues others
Paranoid	Suspicious and blames others for failures
Litigious	Threatens lawsuits and responds to every slight
Compulsive	Preoccupied with orderliness and perfection, intolerant, critical and controlling

Data from Bart, M. (2009). Managing disruptive students in the college classroom. *Faculty Focus*. Retrieved from http://www.facultyfocus.com/articles/effective-classroom-management/managing-disruptive-students-in-the-college-classroom/; Snyder, B. (2010). Coping with seven disruptive personality types in the classroom. *Magna Publications White Paper*. Retrieved from http://www.northwestms.edu/library/Library/Web/magna_wp7.pdf

STUDENTS' AND TEACHERS' RIGHTS AND RESPONSIBILITIES

The rights and responsibilities of students and teachers are usually outlined in the student/faculty handbook of the school where you intend to teach. The handbook may be found as a hard copy or via a link on the school's webpage. It is imperative that you review these rights and responsibilities prior to beginning your appointment and then whenever a question arises. In general, students have the right to a fair and unbiased education.

ACADEMIC INTEGRITY

There are many definitions of academic integrity. In general, academic integrity reflects the values and principles upon which academia is built. It refers to honesty in developing and presenting one's scholarship. Faculty and students alike are expected to present original work or at least to give credit to work that was done by others. One much-discussed breach of academic integrity is plagiarism, which is submitting someone else's work as yours without giving proper credit. With the advancement of technology, creative strategies for plagiarism have expanded into all areas of academe. Why is such an upsurge occurring? Often students are peer-pressured, social-pressured, or self-pressured into cheating. Nursing students have reported a main reason for cheating as being the high-stakes testing that will influence their success or failure and, in most cases, their ability to remain in the nursing program.

Faculty have a right to be preemptive to minimize plagiarism; this includes stating clear policies in the syllabus regarding the consequences of such an act. Such policies also are usually clearly stated in the student/faculty handbook. Plagiarism is not always done intentionally; therefore, it is the faculty's responsibility to explain to students what is considered plagiarism and how to avoid it. The teacher has the responsibility to enforce the rules of academic integrity. Most schools have a policy governing academic integrity. Failing to follow the rules is dealt with in several different ways, ranging from remediation to expulsion from the school.

McCabe and Pavela (2012), researchers on academic integrity, outline the following 10 steps for minimizing breaches in academic integrity:

- Schools should affirm the importance of academic integrity as one of the core values of academia.
- Foster the love of learning in students by making the work challenging, relevant, useful, and fair.
- Treat students respectfully as valued individuals.
- Promote a classroom environment of trust, free of arbitrary rules.
- Hold students accountable for academic integrity. Create fair competitions where integrity is respected and dishonesty or the perception thereof is punished.
- Clarify expectations for students ahead of time and provide guidance in helping students meet their goals.
- Develop and use fair and relevant forms of assessment that promote learning opportunities for students.
- Reduce opportunities to engage in academic dishonesty by removing ambiguous policies, unrealistic standards for collaboration, inadequate classroom management, or poor examination security.
- Challenge academic dishonesty when it occurs by enforcing the stated school policy as a guide.
- Support campus-wide efforts at decreasing academic integrity and standards by identifying students who commit an infraction across campus, especially repeat offenders.

LEARNING COMMUNITIES

The concept of learning communities in colleges has become increasingly popular over the past few years. In a broad sense, learning communities on campus involve a group of students who share similar interests, such as nursing; have common values; live and learn together; and attend a cohort of classes taught by teachers with whom they have close interactions. Whether or not there is such an arrangement on your campus, you may want to consider developing a quasi-learning community for your classes.

Students can be divided into groups based on their interests and learning styles. Clinical faculty can be invited to share in the teaching of these grouped classes. Students' clinical groups will remain constant throughout the semester, with the clinical instructor helping students to meet their individual goals and program outcome. Senior students can be invited to share their experiences as nursing students and give practical advice on how to succeed.

This arrangement gives the students the opportunity to work closely with those who have similar interests as they develop the skills and confidence necessary for future success. Students not only will feel a sense of belonging with their peers and faculty, but also will become more comfortable in seeking advice on their academic achievement and become more comfortable in the school's culture. The overall goal, therefore, would be to have the student succeed socially and academically.

ASSISTING THE ACADEMICALLY CHALLENGED STUDENT

Working with the academically challenged student in the traditional classroom often poses a huge concern for the teacher. Students who are struggling often expect the teacher to spend extra time addressing their needs. In some cases this may not be possible; however, it is the responsibility of the teacher to provide resources that will enhance a student's learning. Depending on the needs of the student, you may refer her or him to several university resources such as a learning center, a writing center, tutoring, or test-taking practice. If the student is struggling with mastering the content, you may want to set aside special office hours time to go over strategies on how to study effectively.

At some point teachers can become frustrated when they believe they are not meeting all of a student's needs. You may also feel conflicted that you have not done enough to assist students in passing exams. It is advisable to discuss these feelings with senior faculty who may have had the same experiences in the past and who may be helpful in providing hints on how to deal with such issues.

CASE STUDY

You are the new pediatric faculty for the Department of Nursing at a local university. You receive your course roster and notice there are 55 students assigned to your section of the course. Your room assignment is S138, the 150-seat amphitheater in the south wing of the building.

1. Create a seating plan to facilitate learning among the students and promote student–teacher relationships.

2. You notice a group of four students sitting in the back of the amphitheater talking and using their cell phones. How would you handle this situation?
3. You are proctoring an exam and notice a student glancing at the answers on another student's test. How would you handle this situation?

REFERENCES

Altmiller, G. (2012). Student perceptions of incivility in nursing education: Implications for educators. *Nursing Education Perspectives, 33*(1), 15–20.

Arieli, D., Mashiach, M., Hirschfeld, M. J., & Friedman, V. (2012). Cultural safety and nursing education in divided societies. *Nursing Education Perspectives, 33*(6), 364–368.

Bart, M. (2009). Managing disruptive students in the college classroom. *Faculty Focus.* Retrieved from http://www.facultyfocus.com/articles/effective-classroom-management/managing-disruptive-students-in-the-college-classroom/

Clark, C. M., & Springer, P. J. (2010). Academic nurse leaders' role in fostering a culture of civility in nursing education. *Journal of Nursing Education, 49*(6), 319–325. doi: 10.3928/01484834-20100224-01. Retrieved from http://www.nsna.org/Portals/0/Skins/NSNA/pdf/Imprint_AprMay08_Feat_Incivility.pdf

Dapremont, J. A. (2014). Black nursing students: Strategies for academic success. *Nursing Education Perspectives, 35*(3), 157–161. doi:10.5480/11-563.1

De Freitas Castro Carrari de Amorim, R., & Da Silva, M. (2014). Nursing faculty's opinion on effectiveness of non-verbal communication in the classroom. *Acta Paulista De Enfermagem, 27*(3), 194–199.

Fowler, M. D. M. (2008). *Guide to the code of ethics for nurses: Interpretation and application.* Silver Spring, MD: American Nurses Association.

Hoffman, R. (2012). Differences in student perceptions of student and faculty incivility among nursing program types: An application of attribution theory (Doctoral dissertation). Retrieved from https://dspace.iup.edu/bitstream/handle/2069/1922/Riah%20Leigh%20Hoffman.pdf?sequence=1

McCabe, D. L., & Pavela, G. (2012). Ten (updated) principles of academic integrity: How faculty can foster student honesty. *Change, 36*(3), 10–15. Retrieved from http://www.jstor.org/stable/40177967

Patrick, H., Ryan, A. M., & Kaplan, A. (2007). Early adolescents' perception of the classroom environment, motivational beliefs, and engagement. *Journal of Educational Psychology, 99*(1), 83–98. Retrieved from https://www.researchgate.net/publication/228364760_

Snyder, B. (Ed.). (2010). Coping with seven disruptive personality types in the classroom. Retrieved from http://www.northwestms.edu/library/Library/Web/magna_wp7.pdf

CHAPTER 6

Evaluation Techniques

OBJECTIVES

- Design a student assignment to measure formative evaluation.
- Design a student assignment to measure summative evaluation.
- Create the evaluation tools you will use to measure formative and summative evaluation strategies.

Nursing programs carry out systematic evaluations designed to determine teaching effectiveness and to measure to what degree predetermined program outcomes have been achieved. Overall, evaluations are used to determine student learning, verify curricular quality, identify areas of challenge, address program improvement, and collect data for reporting to state and other accrediting agencies. Evaluations are carried out by students, faculty, and peers. As explained by the American Association of Colleges of Nursing (AACN, 2013), effective student evaluations provide crucial information about the strengths and weaknesses of a program. Such findings should be used to create substantive changes that ultimately result in better program outcomes.

You will come across two major evaluation strategies used to determine program effectiveness: formative and summative. Formative evaluations are used to monitor students' learning throughout a program. Students' learning is assessed as they progress, feedback is given to the faculty, and changes are made to the curriculum to address these ongoing findings. In other words, faculty utilize student feedback to improve or adjust teaching strategies, leading to improved student outcomes. Formative assessment emphasizes the importance of students' engagement in their own learning. These types of assessments help students identify their strengths and weaknesses. Areas for improvement can then be targeted and addressed by both students and faculty. Such assessments also help faculty identify when students need help and the type of help they need. These needs can be addressed immediately. Formative evaluations are considered low stakes because rarely are final decisions made as a result of these assessments. Examples of formative assessments include quizzes, concept maps, discussions, group work, and feedback on written papers.

Summative evaluations are used at the end of a course or program to determine students' overall learning as well as to determine program effectiveness. Outcomes are measured against predetermined standards and national benchmarks. Examples of summative evaluations include comprehensive final examinations, research papers, final research projects, exit examinations, and Health Education Systems Incorporated

TABLE 6-1 Formative vs. Summative Evaluation Methods	
Formative Evaluation Methods	**Summative Evaluation Methods**
Quizzes	Comprehensive final exams
Concept maps	Research papers
Discussions	Research projects
Group work	Exit examinations
Student feedback	Qualifying exams (e.g., NCLEX, ATI, and EBI)

(HESI) and National Council Licensure Examination (NCLEX) examinations. Summative evaluations are considered high stakes because important decisions such as grade determination, promotion, access to higher levels of education, retention, and continuation in a program are determined by the outcomes. Some teachers have been accused of teaching to the test when assessments are high stakes.

To clarify the differences (see also **Table 6-1**), summative assessments can be regarded as assessments of learning, whereas formative assessments can be regarded as assessments for learning (Looney, 2011).

STANDARDIZED TESTS FOR EVALUATION

You will come in contact with several standardized tests associated with nursing programs. Some are used as admission criteria, others to assess student progress throughout the program, and yet others to evaluate program outcomes and students' ability to successfully pass the NCLEX qualifying examination. In this chapter we will highlight several of the most commonly used standardized tests.

The **Test of Essential Academic Skills (TEAS)** is a basic aptitude test designed to identify students who would succeed in nursing schools and who have the ability to think like a nurse. The test, provided by ATI, is used by some schools as one of the prerequisites for admission into their nursing programs. College students who declare nursing as their major are required to take this test. The test assesses reading, math, science, English, and language usage. Students study for the TEAS on their own using the text and online material. They then complete a proctored online test. Students who fall below a pre-established minimum score for admission will have the opportunity to remediate their performance prior to repeating the test. Some schools allow students to repeat the test only once, whereas other schools allow for a second opportunity. Some schools use the data gathered on these students to design mentoring programs and to put in place strategies to help these students perform well and remain in the nursing program. Students' progress is tracked throughout the program. A major goal in using the TEAS test is to monitor students and decrease attrition rates.

Health Education Systems Incorporated (HESI) is a company that provides tests, commonly known as the HESI exams, and other educational material designed to prepare student nurses for professional licensure and predict their success on tests such as the NCLEX-RN. HESI provides potential nursing students with the opportunity to demonstrate college-level achievement through a program of exams related to undergraduate college courses including math, reading, grammar, vocabulary, and anatomy and physiology. There is also a learning and personality style portion of the exam. There are several different tests, but one of the most commonly used is the Admission Assessment Exam (AAE), which many schools use as an entrance criterion to their nursing programs. The exams are computerized and administered online, and results can be obtained immediately, which is considered a positive aspect of this type of testing. One of the major concerns about these tests is the appropriateness of using them for high-stakes testing. Some schools apply the grade from the HESI as a percentage of the student's final course grade.

Assessment Technologies Institute (ATI) provides a testing program designed to improve student pass rates on the licensing examinations. Students are tested at set periods throughout the nursing program, mainly after specific courses. Students who are unsuccessful at passing an exam have the opportunity to remediate their performance independently or with guidance. With so many opportunities, it is hoped that the student attrition rate will decrease. ATI testing is widely used among several schools nationally, and not surprisingly schools have different ways of implementing the tests from sophomore to senior levels throughout the undergraduate nursing program. These tests help students to prepare more efficiently, increase their confidence, and help them become more familiar with course content and taking online tests such as the NCLEX. The program provides books, DVDs, online practice, and proctored exams. Some schools establish a calendar for when the tests are to be taken based on the course content that is covered, whereas others use the tests as part of formative and summative course and program evaluations. During their final school year students complete content mastery practice exams and a comprehensive predictor assessment test that is designed to gauge the probability of a student's success on the NCLEX. Students also can identify their strengths and weaknesses and review accordingly.

Results are reported in three categories: ATI proficiency levels, the individual scores required to be determined proficient, and the percentage and number of the group at the proficiency level (see **Table 6-2**). There also are reports on individual averages nationally and by programs.

DEVELOPING A TEST BLUEPRINT AND DESIGNING TESTS

As a new faculty member you will find that one of your most important responsibilities is developing test items and administering examinations. Where should you begin?

TABLE 6-2 Sample ATI Reporting		
ATI Proficiency Level	**Individual Score Required to Be Determined Proficient**	**Percentage and Number of Group at Proficiency Level**
Level 3	80.0–100%	10% (5)
Level 2	67.0–79.9%	60% (30)
Level 1	56.0–66.9%	20% (10)
Below Level 1	0.0–55.9%	10% (5)
Data from Educational Benchmarking Inc.		

Start by developing a table of specifications commonly known as a test blueprint or test grid.

A test blueprint is used as a prerequisite to writing an examination. The blueprint is developed as a matrix or chart that includes the test objectives and the number of test items that reflect the content to be tested. The blueprint provides the structure within which the exam is designed and is used to demonstrate psychometric principles in measuring the course objectives. The National Council of State Boards of Nursing (NCSBN) provides a broad overview or set of guidelines that is extremely helpful for first-time developers of test items. This information can be found on the web at www. ncsbn.org/2013_NCLEX_RN_Detailed_Test_Plan_Educator.pdf.

To develop a test blueprint, start by reviewing the course and program objectives to see what outcomes are to be measured, and then consider the types of test questions you plan to include in your exams. Question types can include multiple choice, short answer, case study, true or false, matching, and fill in the blanks. A test blueprint can also include needed skills and clinical performance. Determine the number of questions you plan on using to test a specific set of content, the objectives that are to be tested, and the weight to be given to each objective. By developing a test blueprint you will ensure that all material is tested in the manner you intend.

A sample test blueprint is shown in **Table 6-3**.

Developing the Test Items

As mentioned previously, several test formats can be used to determine course outcomes, including essays or written assignments, short answers, fill in the blanks, multiple choice, true or false, and matching. (The most common form of test questions that you will come across is multiple choice.) Before you begin, review Bloom's taxonomy (discussed in Chapter 3) for cognitive levels of objectives. The content of the test questions should be a mixture of knowledge, comprehension, application, analysis,

TABLE 6-3	Sample Test Blueprint							
Number of content units: 5								
Number of objectives: 5								
Number of questions for the exam: 50								
Level Objectives	**Course Units**		**Obj. 1**	**Obj. 2**	**Obj. 3**	**Obj. 4**	**Obj. 5**
		Number of Questions	15	10	7	6	12
Apply	Unit 1	15	4	3	2	1	5
Demonstrate	Unit 2	10	4	2	1	1	2
Integrate	Unit 3	10	4	2	1	1	2
Create	Unit 4	5	1	1	1	1	1
Evaluate	Unit 5	10	2	2	2	2	2
	Total Questions	**50**					

synthesis, and evaluation. The items should also include a variety of cognitive processes such as cognitive, psychomotor, and affective strategies. Test questions must be aligned to the content objectives. To do this we recommend you develop a test blueprint, as described in the previous section. Test items are based on the knowledge level of the students being taught; for example, junior students may be asked a majority of knowledge and comprehension questions, whereas seniors would be expected to answer more analysis, synthesis, application, and evaluation questions.

Your school may already have created test banks from which you will draw your questions, or you may have to start from scratch and develop your own questions. This can be a very tedious job, especially because test items need to be validated before being placed into general use. Textbook publishers often have an extensive test bank from which you may be able to draw your questions. Check with the publishers of your courses' textbooks to see if they have relevant test banks.

Testing with multiple-choice questions has both advantages and disadvantages (see **Table 6-4**). Some advantages are that the multiple-choice items are objective, they can be used to elicit learning outcomes from a vast amount of content, they can test at different cognitive levels, students must know the content to be successful, and teachers are able to grade the test quite easily. Some disadvantages of multiple-choice questions are that they are difficult to develop and validate, some students have a hard time reading the stems and comprehending the questions, students' frame of

TABLE 6-4 **Advantages and Disadvantages of Testing with Multiple-Choice Questions**

Advantages	Disadvantages
Items are objective.	They are time consuming to develop and validate.
They are easy to administer and score.	Stems or cases can be difficult to read.
They can be used to cover a large amount of content.	Chosen answers may be influenced by students' frame of reference.
They can be used to test several cognitive levels.	Some students may be adept at guessing without knowing the content.
Students must know the content to be successful.	

reference may influence the chosen answers, and if the test developer fails to pay attention to details, students may end up guessing the correct answers without truly knowing the content.

It is not within the scope of this book to delve into how to develop, assemble, administer, and score multiple-choice questions, and establish reliability and validity; however, McDonald (2014) provides a quick review of these processes. **Table 6-5** offers some quick tips to help you develop your test questions and avoid pitfalls.

Here are some sample multiple-choice questions that explain the differences between knowledge-level and higher-order cognitive questioning.

TABLE 6-5 **Tips for Creating Multiple-Choice Questions**

Stems	Options
Provide an adequate amount of information to answer the question.	Keep all options the same length.
Each stem should stand alone and not provide information for a subsequent question.	Be consistent in the use of alphabetical labels or numbers.
Make the content simple and easy to understand.	All options should make sense.
Use action verbs: Avoid the passive voice.	Only one answer should be correct.
Avoid biases of any sort—no names or ethnicity.	Avoid phrases such as "none of the above" and "all of the above."
Include only information that is relevant to the question.	
Use positive voice.	
Avoid the use of age or sex of a patient or client.	

Knowledge-type question:

1. Which of the following statements is the best description of type 1 diabetes? It is a(n)
   a. anabolic disorder in which glucagon levels are decreased and insulin cannot be used by tissues
   b. disease in which there is an impaired ability of the tissues to use insulin
   c. disease of peripheral insulin resistance characterized by beta cell inhibition of insulin
   d. catabolic disorder in which glucagon levels are elevated and insulin is almost absent*

Analysis/synthesis question:

1. A patient is transferred to your unit with reported expressive aphasia and voluntary motor impairment. Based on this report you would suspect that the patient has an injury to the
   a. parietal lobe
   b. occipital lobe
   c. temporal lobe
   d. frontal lobe*

Application-type question:

1. Your patient's ABG report reads as follows: pH $= 7.40$, $PCO_2 = 37$ mm Hg, $HCO_3 = 24$ mEq/L, $PO_2 = 90$ mm Hg. You interpret this as
   a. metabolic acidosis
   b. respiratory acidosis
   c. normal ABG*
   d. respiratory alkalosis

Essay Questions

Essay questions are a popular way of evaluating students' knowledge and ability. Goals of essay questions are to have students demonstrate their writing and comprehension abilities. Each essay question should be specific in its requirements but also should have some opportunities for expressing individual thoughts. Avoid statements in the question that require the student to list things, because this type of question does not give the student the opportunity to demonstrate writing grammatically correct sentences and expressing thoughts or analyzing content.

Essays should be developed so that students can remain focused on what is being asked and not stray too far from the subject requirement. Always provide a rubric with the essay question. A rubric (such as the one in **Table 6-6**) is a scoring tool used

TABLE 6-6 Sample Rubric

Content	Organization and Completeness	Critical Thinking	Writing
5. The writer has an excellent grasp of the content, elaborates fully on the points that are made, and provides comments and new information that contribute to furthering the topic. Gives illustrations and examples.	5. The writing is very well organized, and ideas and information are true and supported by the readings and connected to the question or the issue. The response or answer makes sense. Statements and ideas flow from/to one another. Ideas that support one another are connected.	5. The writing/discussion shows much careful thought and much insight gained about the issue at hand. The writer is able to pose original, interesting questions about the issue(s). Thoughts and conclusions are supported with good reasons.	5. The writing is lively, expressive, and engaging. Word choice is precise and rich. Sentences flow nicely. There are no errors in grammar, punctuation, or spelling.
3. The writer has a moderate grasp of the content, but there are some misunderstandings on the points that are made, and minimal information that contributes to furthering the topic.	3. The writing is moderately organized and makes sense, and some ideas and information are true and supported by the readings and connected to the question or the issue. Statements and ideas flow from one to another and are somewhat connected.	3. The writing/discussion shows some careful thought and insight about most of, but not all, issues. Insights could stand more development. Thoughts and discussions/conclusions could be better supported from the readings.	3. The writing/discussion is pleasant, acceptable, and mostly mechanically correct, but there may still be typographical and spelling errors that interfere with the reading.
1. The writer has only a superficial or fuzzy understanding of the content. There are a number of misunderstandings or false claims that do not contribute to furthering the topic.	1. The writing lacks a coherent structure, and statements and ideas do not flow smoothly from one to another.	1. Not much thought went into the writing/discussion, and there is a lack of interesting or significant insights. Conclusions/ideas are not well supported from the readings.	1. Sentences are choppy, incomplete, rambling, or awkward, or there may be many typographical and spelling errors. Ideas are difficult to comprehend without rereading.

Overall grade scale: 19–20 points = 100; 18–17 points = 90; 16–15 points = 80; 14 or less = 75.

to identify certain criteria within a specific written assignment. Usually rubric grading scores are assigned on a continuum of numbers, letters, or levels of achievement ranked from unsatisfactory to satisfactory, or in the case of nursing from novice to expert. By giving the student the rubric along with the assignment, students are able to review and revise their work prior to submission. They are able to carry out formative and summative evaluations of their work and therefore to clarify their thoughts and judge their own performance.

The following is a sample essay question:

> Describe the function of the cardiac system in the newborn, giving an example of a dysfunctional health pattern. Develop three NANDA nursing diagnoses for this population and their families that include a goal, an intervention, a rationale, and an expected outcome. Discuss five nursing considerations that are critical to the successful outcome in the health of the newborn.

WHAT TO EXPECT AFTER YOU ADMINISTER A TEST

Your work is far from over after you administer the test. Once the results are in, it is imperative that you carry out an item analysis. McDonald (2014) emphasizes the importance of reviewing an exam. Three main goals in reviewing an exam are to

- Identify whether any of the questions are flawed
- Correct any errors and adjust the raw scores
- Improve test items for future use

There are several types of item analysis software on the market, many of which are incorporated into online testing platforms. Results can be obtained instantaneously. Check with your school on how to use them, and attend training if necessary. For a detailed review of how to interpret test results, the following resource is available: *Systematic Assessment of Learning Outcomes: Developing Multiple Choice Questions* (McDonald, 2011).

Do not assign test grades to the exam until you have completed the statistical analysis. You may have to discard flawed items and/or add points to a question that has more than one correct answer. In rare cases you may end up curving the grade; if you have to do so, ensure it is statistically correct to be fair to all students as well as to ensure that the course outcomes are being met.

GRADING

You will no doubt learn quite early in your career how important grades are to students. Grades are a high-stakes representation for the student. They have a social and psychological impact on a student's self-esteem, and in many cases will determine future outcomes. Be fair and accurate. Be willing to discuss with the student how you arrived at the grade. Reviewing an exam in class can be used as a teaching tool, although in some cases this can lead to controversial and even cantankerous classroom behavior. Be prepared to have the rationale for the correct answer to share with students. Bear in mind the overall importance of grades. Once again, we refer you to McDonald (2014) for some grading principles:

- Grades have a significant impact on the lives of students.
- Test items should be congruent with course objectives.
- Strive to use objective grading strategies rather than subjective ones so as to be fair to all students.
- Test items should be reviewed for their validity and reliability as well as for being evidence based.
- Students' privacy must be respected and all scores held in confidence.
- There must be clearly written grading polices that are shared with students early in the semester.
- Grades can be a motivator for students' learning and performance.

Finally, be fully aware of what constitutes a passing or failing grade. Other things to consider prior to testing are whether you will drop a grade, curve an exam, or give students the benefit of the doubt when their scores are on the borderline; how you will react to the school's requirement of a grade spread; whether you have any flexibility in assigning grades; and how you will weight each grade to arrive at a final course grade.

TEST BIAS

Once you have administered your test and completed your item analysis, it is important to take an objective overall look at the test and the results. You may note that there are several variables that impact the test scores, including ethnicity, race, gender, disability, socioeconomic background, ability to speak English, income level, and frame of reference. You will spend a large amount of time designing your tests to avoid bias. It is commonly believed that unfair testing is widespread in academia. As an educator, you must be prepared to defend your assessments against charges of bias. First, be aware of your own biases and keep them out of the academic arena. Fairness is tied closely to validity; for a test to be valid, it must be fair. Bias in testing can and indeed does occur from time to time. As an educator you have the responsibility to minimize bias in testing. Be careful to require only knowledge that is expected of the student. Make sure tests meet their purpose and are appropriate. Avoid racism, sexism, stereotypes, and offensive language. Remember that from the student's point of view, faculty are the subjective dimension to the test. In other words, students often link the test to the nature of the faculty.

Research shows that multiple-choice questions tend to be biased toward males. Multiple-choice questions also seem to be more difficult for students for whom English is their second language. To avoid linguistic structural bias, keep the stems of questions simple and uncomplicated. Avoid lack of clarity, and be consistent in the use of grammar. Finally, review your tests for correctness in structure, punctuation, and spelling.

GRADE APPEAL

Students who believe they have been graded incorrectly have the right to appeal according to established guidelines usually found in the school's student handbook. Should you face such a situation, refer the student to the appeals committee and be prepared to share the student's grade with the committee as well as discuss how the grade was arrived at. A successful appeal of the grade may lead to you either having to readjust the grade or allowing the student to make up the test.

EVALUATIONS

Student Program Evaluation

Program evaluation is the responsibility of students, faculty, and benefactors. Teachers should make every effort to involve their students in assessing all aspects of the program. Students' evaluations can provide crucial input about program effectiveness (McMillan & Shannon, 2011). Students have been shown to be quite adept at evaluating overall program satisfaction in the areas of financial relevance, academic advisement, and quality and rigor of the curriculum. Teachers are encouraged to provide methods for students to evaluate their peers, evaluate the lecture at the end of class, and evaluate the teacher for teaching effectiveness and classroom management. One suggestion for classroom evaluation is having students complete one-sentence statements regarding the class and then submit them for your perusal. This information can then be used to make changes during the next class. With the current use of technology in the classroom you also may want to use online surveys periodically to assess classroom effectiveness.

Faculty Evaluation of Program Effectiveness

It is important that schools carry out periodic evaluations of their programs to determine effectiveness. Schools often review and revise their curricula on a periodic basis to ensure that they are in congruence with national standards and that expected outcomes are being met. There are several established educational standards and competencies that are required to be met for nurses to become certified in their field of practice. It is expected that for a program to be accredited, the standards are met through the program plan and syllabi. Included in overall program evaluation are whether the program outcomes have been met, the graduation rates, the percentage of students who pass the NCLEX on the first try, the graduate employment rate, employer satisfaction with graduates, student satisfaction with the program, and the number of students going on to graduate studies. These data are often obtained through student exit surveys, as well as employer and alumni surveys. Most nursing programs have an evaluation committee that is responsible for collecting and monitoring such data. Accreditation bodies such as ACEN or CCNE require those data to accredit the organization. Recently, accrediting bodies have discussed concerns regarding the poor response to surveys from students and employers. New suggestions for nursing programs are that surveys should be carried out through the use of social media, formation of Facebook groups for graduating classes, and email contact established with students prior to graduation. Programs also need to emphasize to students the importance of responding to the surveys.

According to Story et al. (2010), the following are some innovative ways to improve program evaluation responses to a survey:

- Maximize the use of the web to collect data. It is easy and free.
- Redesign new-employer surveys to be shorter in length (one-page limit).
- Send the surveys to the human resources director rather than the nurse administrator.
- Eliminate paper and pencil surveys, which yield a poor response.
- Reach out to alumni through online social networks.
- Develop effective ways to communicate with alumni through email.

Peer Evaluation

The overall goal of peer evaluation is to promote excellence in educational practices. However, peer evaluation is another one of those contentious issues for faculty. Often, more seasoned faculty do not appreciate being scrutinized by either newer faculty or their peers. For effective faculty evaluation to be carried out, administrative intervention to ensure peer review must be established in the framework of the institution. These guidelines are put in place to ensure that peer evaluation occurs and that the results are analyzed and documented according to policy. It has been suggested by the Center for Teaching Excellence (CTE) that administrative intervention is necessary to ensure peer evaluation has occurred. As a new faculty member, it is advisable to have your peers evaluate your classroom performance so that you can make substantive adjustments to your teaching and classroom management. When properly carried out, peer evaluation can help you avoid the pitfalls arising from student evaluations.

The multiple purposes of peer evaluation include the following:

- *Formative:* To develop or improve teaching effectiveness and student learning
- *Summative:* To provide documentation of teaching effectiveness for formal review and career advancement, or tenure

Each peer reviewer brings a different kind of experience and expertise to the process. Therefore, which colleague is appropriate to choose as a peer evaluator depends on the purpose of the review.

CASE STUDIES

1. Your course is in the fourth week of the semester and you have been teaching about the concept of circulation. You want to evaluate students' understanding of this concept and how alterations in this concept may affect the health of their patients. Design a student assignment that will help you evaluate students' understanding of how alterations in this concept affect the health of their patient.
2. You are developing the final exam for your level-two nursing course. The final exam will consist of 50 multiple choice questions. Develop a test blueprint with five multiple choice questions to measure your stated course objectives. Be sure each question addresses one of the five levels of Bloom's taxonomy.

REFERENCES

Billings, D. M., & Halstead, J. A. (2012). *Teaching in nursing: A guide for faculty* (4th ed.).St. Louis, MO: Elsevier.

Looney, J. W. (2011, April). Integrating formative and summative assessment: Progress toward a seamless system? *OECD Education Working Papers,* 58.

McDonald, M. (2011). *Systematic assessment of learning outcomes: Developing multiple choice questions* (3rd ed.). Burlington, MA: Jones & Bartlett Learning.

McDonald, M. (2014). *The nurse educator's guide to assessing learning outcomes* (3rd ed.). Burlington, MA: Jones & Bartlett Learning.

McMillan, L. R., & Shannon, D. (2011). Program evaluation of nursing school instruction in measuring students' perceived competence to empathetically communicate with patients. *Nursing Education Perspectives, 32*(3), 150–154. Retrieved from http://dx.doi.org.library2.ramapo.edu:2048/10.5480/1536-5026-32.3.150

Clinical Teaching

CHAPTER 7

Contextual Factors Influencing the Clinical Experience

OBJECTIVES

- Explain how a school of nursing's mission, philosophy, and program outcomes guide the development of the curriculum and clinical objectives.
- Identify factors faculty need to consider when preparing to use a clinical agency and your responsibilities in ensuring these factors are met.
- Explain the various clinical teaching models available and faculty's roles in each model.
- Appraise the appropriateness of clinical agencies for helping students satisfy clinical objectives.

The sweeping changes occurring in the healthcare environment, coupled with the increased multiculturalism of society, expanding technology, a critical shortage of nurse educators, and mandates from the federal government for the accountability of student learning outcomes by schools of higher education, have called for new ways of teaching. This need is evident in the clinical preparation of nursing students who are being educated to work in our changing healthcare environment. As educators, it is our responsibility to prepare our nursing students with clinical experiences that will help them be ready to deliver safe nursing care to individuals with complex healthcare needs across the lifespan.

As a nurse educator in academia, your teaching responsibilities extend beyond the walls of the classroom to clinical agencies in the community. These clinical agencies provide the environment in which students apply the knowledge of the nursing process they have gained through classroom teaching. Clinical agencies may include acute care hospitals, rehabilitation centers, assisted and long-term care facilities, outpatient centers, and clinics. Because these clinical agencies serve many different healthcare needs of patients, providing students with experiences in these environments gives them an opportunity to apply their knowledge of nursing across the health and wellness continuum. Exposure to these differing healthcare settings allows students to experience the multifaceted roles and responsibilities of professional nurses while helping them to develop in their future roles.

Depending on the nursing program where you are employed, you may be responsible for the didactic delivery of course content in the classroom while other faculty, hired as clinical instructors or preceptors, are responsible for students' learning experiences in the clinical setting. Regardless of the scope of your teaching responsibilities, faculty need to be very familiar with the contextual factors that may influence students' clinical experiences. These factors include the nursing program's mission, philosophy, and program outcomes as well as clinical selection criteria and the appropriateness, availability, and types of clinical agencies.

NURSING PROGRAM'S MISSION, PHILOSOPHY, AND OUTCOMES

The nursing program's mission, philosophy, and outcomes guide the development of the curriculum and influence the nurse educator's selection of clinical sites, clinical objectives, and learning experiences. The nursing program's mission statement informs the public of its purpose—why it exists, who it intends to serve, and the standards to which the school aspires. The nursing program philosophy identifies the values and beliefs of the school as they relate to beliefs about nursing, learning, and nursing education (Billings & Halstead, 2016). Program outcomes are the knowledge, skills, and abilities nursing students should possess when they graduate from a nursing program. The nurse educator needs to understand and espouse the school's mission, philosophy, and learning outcomes to provide the most relevant clinical experiences that will help nursing students develop in their professional role.

The nursing program's mission, philosophy, and outcomes will vary depending on the level of the degree program; for example, in a two-year associate degree or four-year baccalaureate degree the program outcome may be to graduate students who are prepared as safe, beginning-level registered nurses. In contrast, in a graduate nursing program the outcome may be to graduate registered nurses who are prepared for advanced practice roles in the healthcare system. Regardless of the type of nursing program and the nursing degree awarded to students, there are several factors faculty need to consider when selecting clinical assignments.

CLINICAL CONTRACT AND AGENCY REQUIREMENTS

The curriculum in all nursing programs involves classroom and clinical learning experiences. For schools of nursing to provide clinical experiences for their students, the college or university needs to have contractual agreements with the various healthcare settings where students' clinical experiences are anticipated to occur. These contracts clearly identify the roles and responsibilities of the school of nursing and its faculty who come to the clinical site. Clinical agency contracts are legally binding documents created between the college's legal counsel and the agency's administration. These contracts clearly define the rights and responsibilities of each involved party.

The clinical agency retains full responsibility for the care of the patients and will maintain collaborative responsibility with the college or university for the supervision of students and faculty to the extent their presence may affect the operation of the clinical agency and care of the patients. The clinical agency has the right to suspend a student from utilizing the clinical agency for clinical experience if the clinical agency experiences any situation where a student's performance is unsatisfactory. This cooperative agreement between the clinical agency and the school of nursing does not include financial compensation to either party. The clinical agency will provide an orientation for faculty and students to explain the rules, regulations, and procedures of the facility when deemed necessary.

The college or university assumes full responsibility for the planning, scheduling, and execution of the educational experiences provided by qualified nursing instructors and shares these schedules with the clinical agency. The college or university ensures all faculty and students have malpractice insurance and health clearance, including documented proof of immunizations, prior to the start of the clinical experience. Faculty and students are also required to have any specialized training deemed necessary by the agency before placement in the facility for educational experiences. Faculty and students are expected to abide by the rules of the agency regarding the confidentiality of all medical and personnel information and any other agency policies and procedures related to the delivery of patient care (U.S. Department of Health and Human Services, n.d.).

LEARNER NEEDS AND PROGRAM OUTCOMES

When clinical sites are chosen for student clinical experiences, the learners' needs and the program outcomes will influence that choice. If students are enrolled in a nursing program to obtain an associate or baccalaureate degree, initially you may want to consider a clinical site where patients have simple nursing needs such as bathing, toileting, feeding, medication administration, and communication. Because students are expected to implement these nursing needs in a safe and knowledgeable manner, placing students in this environment may help them begin to feel more comfortable with their delivery of nursing care while experiencing firsthand the roles and responsibilities of the nurse. Ironically, during this initial exposure to patient care some students come to realize that nursing is not their preferred career and may withdraw from the nursing program. Other students become exhilarated with their nursing care assignments and continue on with confidence and determination to be successful and graduate from nursing school.

As students progress through the nursing curriculum, they continue to learn about patients with more complex needs. Students can then be assigned to clinical sites where patients have more complex needs such as dressing changes, suctioning, tube feedings, and patient teaching. Students are now assigned clinical experiences that will give them the opportunity to apply this more advanced nursing knowledge. Prelicensure programs are designed to progressively develop students in their nursing knowledge and clinical skills, so the choice of students' clinical assignments will depend on how much learning they have acquired at the time when they are assigned a clinical placement. When faculty choose clinical assignments for nursing students, they need to take into consideration the nursing course that students are presently taking and the objectives for that course. For example, if students are enrolled in a community health course and have already completed a course in adult health, faculty may want to consider sending students to a community health clinic for diabetic patients.

In a graduate nursing program designed to prepare registered nurses for advanced practice roles, students together with their faculty may need to find clinical placements that promote attainment of course objectives. For example, if a registered nurse has chosen to prepare for the advanced practice role with a specialty in gerontology, that nurse may seek clinical experiences with a geriatric population in an adult care center or long-term facility. Once again, the course syllabus together with course objectives and learner outcomes are carefully reviewed by faculty to help ensure the needed alignment between classroom learning and clinical assignments prior to approving the student's choice of clinical placement. All necessary clinical affiliation contracts need to be established between the college or university and the approved clinical agency.

RELATIONSHIP WITH THE CLINICAL AGENCY AND STAFF

Another criterion for faculty to consider when selecting clinical experiences is the relationship with the clinical agency and the staff. Some clinical agencies and staff are very willing to have students come to their facility for learning experiences, whereas other agencies are not. If the school of nursing already has a contract with the agency, this means the agency has agreed to have students come to the facility.

The clinical environment is a place where students synthesize the knowledge gained in the classroom and apply this knowledge to practical situations. Regardless of the location of the clinical assignment, faculty and agency staff should provide an environment where students are made to feel welcome and are appreciated for their contributions to patient care.

Clinical nursing faculty are licensed practitioners and therefore able to practice or teach nursing only in a state where they are licensed. For this reason, agencies used as clinical sites need to be selected according to where nursing faculty hold licensure. At times, especially in distance education graduate nursing programs, a clinical agency may be appropriate for meeting students' learning needs but there are no faculty from the school of nursing who hold licensure in the state where the clinical agency is located. In this case, the school of nursing and the agency may need to establish specific regulations regarding who will be responsible for providing students with the clinical experiences needed to satisfy course objectives using this distance placement method. Some distance placement clinical agencies may have designated nursing staff as preceptors to serve the learning needs of nursing students from out-of-state schools of nursing. In this situation, the clinical agency and the school of nursing will have clinical contracts identifying the responsibilities of both parties for meeting the educational needs of the students.

Clinical placements of students in the same state where the school of nursing is located are often a collaborative effort between the clinical agency and faculty. Faculty are often familiar with the various clinical agencies in the state and have established relationships with the staff from these agencies. Faculty are aware of the learning experiences available at these agencies and meet with the agency staff to plan and organize students' clinical placements. Agencies and schools of nursing use several different models for student clinical assignments; these models are discussed in more detail later in this chapter. Some clinical agencies may adhere to a model requiring faculty from the school of nursing to be present at all times when students are at the agency, whereas other agencies may use a preceptor model to facilitate students' clinical experiences.

LOCATION OF THE CLINICAL AGENCY

In addition to choosing clinical sites in certain state jurisdictions, the geographic location of the school of nursing may be considered. Students should not be expected to travel a long distance from the school of nursing to their clinical sites. Usually colleges try to keep the travel distance to a clinical site within a reasonable number of miles from the school. For a prelicensure program, in most cases local clinical placements will be assigned within the state jurisdiction of the school of nursing and faculty licensure.

In contrast, clinical placements in a graduate nursing program may expand beyond the state jurisdiction of the school of nursing. This often occurs when the graduate nursing program is delivered through distance education and online learning.

A student enrolled in an online nursing graduate program may hold licensure from a state different from the state where the school is located. In this case, schools of nursing allow their graduate students to pursue clinical placements in agencies close to their home and do not require students to travel to the state where the school of nursing is located. Often with these distance placement clinical experiences, graduate students find their own preceptors. In graduate nursing programs that allow students to find their own clinical preceptors, contractual agreements are established outlining faculty, student, and preceptor responsibilities to ensure course objectives and clinical hours are satisfied. All preceptors must be approved by the school of nursing and meet the necessary qualifications of a clinical instructor. In most cases, these preceptors are not financially compensated by the school of nursing. Because some states may require students in any clinical learning environment to obtain an RN licensure in their states, students who pursue clinical placement outside their state licensure are usually responsible for contacting the state's nursing board to find out the licensure requirements for out-of-state clinical experiences.

AVAILABILITY OF ROLE MODELS

When students are assigned to various clinical agencies for their clinical experience, faculty need to consider several different factors about the nursing staff presently employed in the selected agency. Nursing students may perceive nursing staff as role models and may often imitate their behaviors. As role models, these nurses may contribute to mentoring of these students as beginning or advanced practice nurses. When selecting clinical sites, faculty awareness of nursing staff personalities and characteristics can contribute to students' learning experiences. Nursing staff should be up-to-date with both their nursing care knowledge and the policies and procedures of the agency. As good mentors, they should be willing to take time out of their busy day to interact with the students and be committed to actively participating in students' learning (Ali & Panther, 2008). When staff are good mentors, they are willing to share their skills, knowledge, and expertise with the students. They demonstrate a positive attitude toward their work responsibilities and administer nursing care in a calm, friendly manner despite the stressors that may surround them. They are compassionate toward students, understand and respect learner differences, and strive to empower students to develop their own strengths, beliefs, and personal attributes. They provide the guidance and constructive feedback required to help students identify their own strengths and weaknesses while planning for student growth in the clinical setting.

Good mentors are good communicators. They can communicate with students in a nonjudgmental way while providing the positive reinforcement and encouragement students need to enhance their self-confidence. Good mentors maintain frequent communication with faculty regarding student progress and are willing to provide feedback for student clinical evaluations.

Clinical faculty need to establish close working relationships with agency staff assigned to students' clinical experiences. In a sense, this relationship will complement your role as clinical faculty.

FACULTY EXPERTISE IN CLINICAL TEACHING

Now that you have decided to be a faculty member in a nursing program, you need to know how to teach. Knowing how to teach in the clinical setting to foster progressive development of your students requires you to be aware of some fundamental facts about teaching in the clinical setting. Being the expert clinician you are is not enough to ensure you can teach effectively in the clinical setting. As a clinical educator you need to know how to assess student learning needs and plan teaching strategies to meet these needs and satisfy course objectives and student learning outcomes. The clinical area provides you with the place to develop and implement these teaching strategies. (These teaching strategies will be discussed in more depth in Chapter 9.) In addition to having a working knowledge of teaching strategies, you need to understand some basic responsibilities needed by faculty to be effective in the clinical setting.

An effective clinical teacher creates the environment needed to guide students' learning experiences in the clinical setting. This requires knowledge of the teaching/learning process such that you become the facilitator of learning and the student is an active participant in that learning process. Clinical teaching is a time when your students are given the opportunity to apply the nursing process to patient care with you there as a resource person. Clinical teaching is not the time for you, the expert clinician, to show your students your skills and tell them how to perform nursing care.

Box 7-1 Effective Clinical Educators

Effective clinical educators...
- create a learning environment.
- are knowledgeable about course objectives and student learning outcomes.
- identify student learning needs.
- are aware of student characteristics.
- are able to guide students through difficult times.
- evaluate students' clinical performance and provide timely feedback.
- ask thought-provoking, open-ended questions to stimulate critical thinking.
- know who they are as educators.

Instead, it should be a time when students take on the responsibility to apply what they have learned in the classroom and laboratory to the care of their patients with you available as a resource person with information to share if needed. Remember, teaching is not telling; it is not demonstrating your skills. Instead, teaching is involving students as active participants in their clinical learning experiences (Gaberson & Oermann, 2010).

An effective clinical teacher is knowledgeable about course objectives and student learning outcomes. These intended learning outcomes often set the direction for students' experiences in the clinical area. There is an expectation that students will achieve progressive competencies as they proceed through the nursing program. Once you are aware of these competencies and expected student outcomes, you can plan for clinical experiences that will give students the opportunity to progressively develop in their roles as beginning or advanced practitioners. Clinical competencies usually center on the student's knowledge of the pathophysiology of the disease; the implementation of the nursing process in the delivery of care; the quality and safety of health care; communication with patients, families, and the healthcare team; and self-development including leadership abilities, accountability, and continued learning. In other words, these competencies address the cognitive, affective, and psychomotor domains of the learning process presented in previous chapters in this book.

At times you may find some students are unable to achieve certain competencies. At this point you will use your expertise to identify student learning needs and possible reasons why they are unable to achieve the expected course outcomes needed for them to progressively develop in the delivery of their nursing care. When assessing student learning needs, you determine whether students have learned the prerequisite knowledge and skills needed to perform the task at hand. It is at this point you are making the determination of whether students are able to transfer classroom content and laboratory experiences to the clinical setting. Keep in mind that not every student is able to transfer these learnings to the clinical setting with the same expected competency. Students may need additional coaching from you to correctly perform the task at hand. The clinical setting provides an excellent environment for you to provide the coaching students may need to move forward in their learning. However, as clinical faculty you need to determine how much coaching students should receive before they are evaluated as unable to meet expected outcomes. At times this is a difficult decision for the inexperienced clinical faculty member to make. This brings us to another important factor for you to be aware of in the process of clinical teaching—the characteristics of the learner.

Some students have the self-determination to succeed and overcome the challenges that come with attending a nursing program. They spend long hours reading, studying, and preparing for their clinical assignments. Others are less dedicated in their pursuit of education. Faculty need to understand these student differences and attempt to help students identify their limitations and what they need to do to achieve success in the nursing program.

An effective clinical teacher has the ability to guide students through their learning experiences. Some students may require more guidance than others. When we guide students to learn from their clinical experiences, we provide a supportive process that helps students achieve the expected outcomes. This supportive process begins with creating an atmosphere of trusting relationships between students and faculty that supports open communication, encourages students to explore alternatives, and recognizes students' accomplishments with constructive feedback. This relationship between faculty and students is one where students feel faculty care about their ability to succeed. Faculty are available to provide students with support, especially when some students are having difficulty transferring their nursing knowledge and skills to the clinical setting. Students need to feel that faculty are friends and mentors rather than adversaries.

Effective clinical educators are able to evaluate students' clinical performances and provide timely feedback on students' progress without degrading their confidence. Faculty also provide students with opportunities to evaluate their own clinical performance. By maintaining close observation of students' abilities to implement nursing care in a safe, knowledgeable manner, faculty are able to identify students' strengths and weaknesses and plan for future clinical experiences. Communicating these strengths and weaknesses to students may be challenging for the inexperienced educator. Informing students of their strengths is an easy process for both experienced and inexperienced educators because students feel good about themselves and are receptive to this feedback from faculty. However, informing students of their weaknesses is not feedback that is easy for inexperienced faculty to give. When students receive negative feedback and their weaknesses are identified, they are often unreceptive to this information and become defensive in their responses. Inexperienced faculty often are uncomfortable with this reaction from students. Ironically, it is this feeling of discomfort that prevents faculty from providing the guidance students need to improve. Inexperienced faculty would rather avoid confronting students with their limitations than provide students with the guidance they need to overcome their weaknesses. If students are to achieve progressive development in the clinical area, they must be told of their weaknesses and provided with the help they need from faculty to overcome these weaknesses. Faculty who do not tell students of their weaknesses deprive students of the opportunity to develop professionally in their nursing roles. As an inexperienced educator, you need to believe this and not resist discussing students' weaknesses with them. After all, everything you do as an educator is intended to enhance student learning and success.

An effective clinical educator is able to ask thought-provoking, open-ended questions that stimulate critical thinking in students. Questions asked by faculty need to help students hone their decision-making and problem-solving skills. Often when faculty ask these types of questions, students begin to feel intimidated by this kind of questioning. Faculty need to make students aware of why they are using such questioning—namely, to help them develop critical thinking skills. Explaining this rationale to students often alleviates their feelings of inadequacy, and they feel more comfortable when responding to faculty questions. By using this form of questioning, faculty gain some insight into students' ability to think critically in the clinical setting. It is our responsibility as clinical educators to prepare future nurses to use critical thinking when providing patient care. The clinical setting is one place where this competency can be encouraged and achieved.

Finally, effective clinical educators know who they are as educators, their values and beliefs about students and education, and any biases they hold that may cloud their evaluation of students. As new clinical faculty you may not have had enough experiences to fully solidify your values and beliefs about the roles and responsibilities of the nurse educator and the student. Just as your values and beliefs about nursing have developed over time from your experiences in health care, so, too, will your values and beliefs about education and students develop over time.

CLINICAL TEACHING MODELS

Healthcare agencies and schools of nursing currently use several clinical teaching models when preparing for students' clinical assignments. Clinical faculty need to be familiar with the different clinical teaching models and work with agencies and their staff to implement these models to ensure student learning and achievement of course objectives. The choice of which clinical model an agency and nursing program will use may depend on various factors such as availability of qualified nursing faculty, the patient acuity level, the number of assigned students and their skill level, and clinical agency resources including the availability of staff and technology. The shortage of qualified nurse educators coupled with the increasing enrollment of students into prelicensure and graduate-level programs has challenged schools of nursing to rethink the ways in which clinical education is provided to students. Working together with clinical agencies, schools of nursing have begun to evaluate the effectiveness of the different clinical teaching models for student learning experiences and achievement of student outcomes.

The traditional model for student clinical placement is one where students are taught in a clinical setting by faculty from the nursing program. This model is often used in prelicensure nursing programs with student-to-faculty ratios ranging from 1:8 to 1:10. Patients are selected based on course objectives and students' level in the program. Students may be assigned to one or two patients and assume responsibility for the nursing care they give to their patients. Under the guidance of the faculty, the students implement the nursing process learned in the classroom as they assess, plan, implement, and evaluate their patients' health status and nursing care needs. At times, if patients have complex nursing needs, faculty may consider assigning two students to the same patient. This helps build collaboration and communication among the students, may decrease students' anxiety levels, and may decrease the number of patients for whom the faculty member is responsible. This traditional model requires faculty to be present with the students on the clinical unit while directly overseeing the nursing care delivered by the students.

In graduate nursing programs, nursing faculty do not need to directly supervise the learning experiences of the students as they do in prelicensure programs because students in graduate programs already have licenses as registered nurses. The traditional model is not appropriate for creating clinical assignments in graduate nursing programs because faculty cannot be present at all times during these clinical assignments. Students enrolled in a graduate nursing program have different learning needs based on their choice of a specific advanced practice role and will require many different clinical placements. In this case, faculty may visit the clinical site only as needed to determine if students are meeting course objectives. In the absence of clinical faculty, specific agency staff may provide for the clinical learning needs of the graduate student. Agency staff may include physicians or other advanced practice nurses who act as mentors or preceptors for the graduate student. In such cases, contracts between the school of nursing and the clinical agency will identify the roles and responsibilities of all parties involved.

Another model for clinical assignments is the preceptor model. This model is appropriate for prelicensure and graduate nursing programs and helps bridge the gap between the classroom and the clinical area (Shpritz & O'Mara, 2006). The faculty member functions as the liaison between the preceptor, the student, and the clinical site. The faculty member works closely with the preceptor to provide an orientation to the preceptor role, course objectives, and student outcomes. This orientation may include information about clinical teaching techniques, communication and conflict resolution, management of the clinical learning environment, supervision, and evaluation of students. Preceptors are also made aware of the policies and procedures of the school of nursing. Two-way communication is maintained between the faculty and the preceptor as well as between the faculty and the student throughout the clinical assignment. Faculty are available to the preceptor and the students in various ways—for example, by scheduled visits to the clinical site, telephone communication, and emails.

The preceptor is an experienced registered nurse with clinical expertise in the area of student needs and course objectives. Preceptors are selected for their level of education, clinical knowledge, and desire to teach. The level of education required to be a preceptor for nursing students in the clinical area will depend on the qualifications set forth by the school of nursing and state board of nursing. For example, to precept in a prelicensure program, preceptors may need to have a baccalaureate or master's degree in nursing, whereas in graduate nursing programs the preceptor may need to have a minimum of a master's or doctorate degree in addition to certification as an advanced practice nurse.

Preceptors, through their role modeling, help prepare student nurses with the variety of skills they will need to function as entry-level or advanced practice nurses. Course objectives and student learning outcomes help the preceptor assess the learning needs of the students. Working collaboratively with the student and faculty, the preceptor identifies clinical experiences that may meet the students' learning outcomes and guides the students in their selection of clinical experiences. While at the clinical site, the preceptor helps students acquire the skills needed to individualize nursing care and solve problems. Preceptors assess students' ability to manage clinical assignments and provide positive and negative feedback to students about their patient care. In situations where students may require more direct supervision on more complex problems, the preceptor is available to help these students acquire the additional knowledge and skills needed for the attainment of course objectives and student learning outcomes. Throughout the clinical assignment, the preceptor keeps the faculty abreast of students' progress in the clinical area. If a student is not advancing in her or his ability to deliver nursing care in a safe and knowledgeable way, the preceptor, student, and faculty will meet to discuss the student's limitations while developing a plan for progressive improvement. At the end of the clinical rotation, the preceptor and faculty validate the student's ability to meet course objectives.

Academic–practice partnerships between schools of nursing and clinical agencies are another model used in clinical education. This concept of partnership to support nursing education was first documented in 1999 by the American Association of Colleges of Nursing (AACN) in *Essential Clinical Resources for Nursing's Academic Mission* (AACN, 2016). This publication explored the need for innovative and effective clinical teaching models that extended beyond the traditional clinical education model historically in place, with the hope of leading to new opportunities for nursing education. It was not until publication of the Institute of Medicine's 2010 report, *The Future of Nursing: Leading Change, Advancing Health*, and the resulting formation of the American Association of Colleges of Nursing–American Origination of Nurse Executives (AACN-AONE) task force on academic–practice partnerships, that this clinical model for nursing education made headway on how clinical education could be improved between schools of nursing and clinical agencies. These academic–practice partnerships are thought to be an important mechanism to strengthen nursing practice while creating systems for nurses to acquire the educational requirements for career advancement, lifelong learning, and residency programs designed to advance the role of the nurse in providing for the health of the public (Beal, 2012).

Underlying these academic–practice partnerships are guiding principles to foster relationships between academia and practice settings that allow for the educational and career advancement needs of nurses while addressing the recommendations set forth by the IOM's Future of Nursing Committee. These principles include the following:

- Establish collaborative relationships between academic and practice settings that have shared vision and mutual goals for the role of the nurse in this changing healthcare system.
- Ensure there is transparency between these two groups, which should be united with respect and trust, joint accountability, mutual investment, commitment, and affirmation to resolve conflict.
- Ensure knowledge is shared between the two groups aimed at enhancing lifelong learning among faculty and practitioners. This knowledge is shared through joint research, committee appointments, preparation for national certifications, and the unfolding and utilization of current best practices.
- Ensure both partners are committed to maximizing the potential of registered nurses to reach their highest level within their scope of practice. There is a shared responsibility to provide opportunities for nurses to lead change efforts in the profession that advocate for the healthcare needs of the public.
- Make a shared commitment to develop a sustainable, cost-effective, evidence-based transition program. This may be the development of residency programs for new graduates and advanced practitioner students.
- Create organizational structures between the partners that recognize and support academic or educational achievements. This can be accomplished by developing seamless academic programs in undergraduate and graduate schools of nursing that allow nurses to advance to their highest level of practice. Both partners recognize and support the need for achieving an 80 percent baccalaureate-prepared RN workforce and for doubling the number of nurses with doctoral degrees. Funding for these programs is a shared responsibility between academia and the practice setting. Grant money and tuition reimbursements are some means to obtain the financial support needed.
- Create collaborative models to redesign nursing education and practice environments. This may involve the formation of joint faculty appointments and joint mentoring programs between academia and clinical agencies.
- Make a joint commitment to collect and analyze data on the current and future needs of the RN workforce. This would include following trends in the healthcare system to determine where the RN workforce can best be utilized to promote health and wellness in society (AACN, 2012; Institute of Medicine, 2010).

Several university schools of nursing have begun to address this need for academic–practice partnerships. As this model gains momentum, nursing education will move forward to design and implement the changes needed to prepare the next generation of professional nurses. It will take years of dedication, commitment, and shared responsibilities between academia and practice settings to help this model come to fruition.

One model for nursing clinical education that evolved from academic–practice partnerships is the Dedicated Education Unit (DEU) (Moscato et al., 2007), which was developed to create an optimal teaching/learning environment for students enrolled in baccalaureate nursing programs. Through collaborative efforts among management in clinical agencies, academic faculty, and clinical nursing staff, the DEU is designated as a special client unit designed to provide opportunities for students to learn in a receptive and nurturing environment by capitalizing on the expertise of both clinical nursing staff and faculty who provide training for the nursing staff on the DEU. Similar to the preceptor model, students are given opportunities to work one-on-one with staff nurses, who have been prepared at minimum at the BSN level. These staff nurses function as clinical instructors or preceptors who provide opportunities for students to experience a realistic picture of nursing practice. The faculty from the school of nursing serve as clinical faculty coordinators who mentor or coach the nursing staff in their roles as clinical instructors. This partnership between faculty and clinical instructors creates a synergistic environment that maximizes student learning outcomes and helps faculty remain current in clinical reality, while also helping nurses develop in their teaching role.

Another clinical education model resulting from academic–practice partnerships is residency programs for new graduates from baccalaureate or graduate nursing programs (Goode et al., 2009). In 2000, the University Health System Consortium (UHC) and the AACN worked collaboratively to develop strategies to address the nursing shortage and prepare new graduates with the expertise required to meet the workforce needs of the changing healthcare environment. From these efforts emerged a formal curriculum for nurse residency programs. These one-year programs exist in approximately 30 states throughout the United States (UHC & AACN, 2016). The programs are built on an evidence-based curriculum designed to provide graduate nurses with learning and work experiences to help them transition into their first professional positions in the acute care setting. The UHC/AACN has a nurse residency program product offering that may be purchased by clinical organizations that want to develop residency programs in their facilities (UHC & AACN, 2008).

TYPES OF CLINICAL AGENCIES

Many different types of clinical agencies can be used by nursing programs for student clinical placements; however, prior to placing students in a clinical setting, faculty need to assess the appropriateness of the clinical site for helping students meet course objectives. Faculty need to be familiar with the agency's culture and structure. Is this agency receptive to student placements, and is it willing to make accommodations for students to enhance their learning experiences? Are agency staff functioning within their scope of practice, and do they have the clinical expertise necessary to function as role models for students? Are agency policies and procedures current with professional practice? Are sufficient equipment and supplies available to students to help them meet the clinical objectives? Are there any reports from regulatory or accreditation surveys that are of concern and may interfere with students' ability to meet the course objectives?

Aside from asking those critical questions about the culture and organization of the agencies, faculty need to be concerned about the clinical experiences available to students in these agencies and identify how these clinical experiences will support the curriculum by aligning with course objectives and student learning outcomes. Faculty need to determine which clinical areas are available for students' learning experiences as well as the acuity level of patients. What are the staffing patterns on these clinical units and are they sufficient to establish a productive teaching/learning environment? Are there nurses who possess the characteristics of role models? Are there opportunities for interdisciplinary activities to complement and expand students' learning experiences?

Once faculty can answer these questions with some degree of certainty, there are various healthcare settings in which faculty may choose to place their students for clinical rotations. Clinical placement settings may include acute care facilities, rehabilitation centers, chronic or long-term care facilities, and ambulatory settings such as outpatient clinics. Quite often faculty choice of clinical agencies will depend on whether the school of nursing is an undergraduate- or graduate-level program.

Acute care hospitals are the clinical agencies used most often by nursing undergraduate and graduate programs. These agencies offer students the opportunity to apply the nursing process across developmental stages with a variety of patients with different healthcare problems and varying acuity levels. Because hospitals are designed to provide for the healthcare needs of patients during the acute stage of illness, students have the opportunity to plan for and experience the delivery of complex nursing skills.

There are several different types of rehabilitation centers offering short- and long-term care to patients. Short-term rehabilitation centers have extensive programs for patients following their posthospital care in areas including orthopedic, cardiovascular, neurological, and postsurgery. Depending on the needs of the patient, physical, occupational, and speech therapy and pain management may also be available at these short-term rehabilitation centers. The goal of these short-term rehabilitation centers, sometimes referred to as subacute centers, is to provide for the continuing healthcare needs of patients while helping them return to their maximum level of wellness.

Sometimes patients in subacute settings do not reach a level of wellness that allows them to return home, such that they need to be placed in chronic or long-term care facilities. There are also substance abuse rehabilitation centers with services aimed at assisting individuals and their families who are struggling with alcohol and drug addiction problems. Some short-term centers may also provide hospice services for patients with terminal medical illnesses.

Chronic or long-term care facilities provide skilled nursing care and/or custodial care for patients with chronic medical problems, permanent disabilities, dementia, or continuous need for help with activities of daily living. Patients in these facilities become residents for an extended period of time and rarely return home. These long-term care facilities provide living accommodations for the residents, who are predominantly members of the geriatric population and require professional health services and personal care including meals, laundry, and housekeeping.

Ambulatory care is medical and nursing care that does not require an overnight stay in a hospital and is provided in such locations as medical offices, clinics, and health departments. The goal of ambulatory care is to maintain wellness and prevent disease among the patient population. This community-oriented clinical practice offers the foundation for community and public health nursing.

When selecting from the various types of clinical agencies for student learning, faculty need to keep in mind whether the nursing program's mission is to prepare students for an undergraduate or graduate nursing degree, the learning objectives of the clinical experience, students' knowledge and skills levels, and the desired student learning outcomes. In addition to applying the necessary nursing skills, students need to develop those problem-solving, decision-making, critical-thinking, and clinical-reasoning skills required of nurses in any healthcare setting. Therefore, when selecting from these various healthcare environments to provide learning experiences for nursing students, faculty need to ensure that clinical learning activities are structured so that they relate logically and sequentially to desired student outcomes (Gaberson & Oermann, 2015).

SUMMARY

This chapter identified the various types of clinical agencies that may be used for nursing student clinical education. The criteria faculty need to consider when choosing a clinical agency for student learning were also addressed. The chapter also identified faculty characteristics you need to enhance your ability to be an effective clinical educator. Finally, the various clinical teaching models used by schools of nursing to provide clinical education to their students were presented. The clinical faculty role in each of these models was described.

CASE STUDIES

1. You are newly hired as a clinical instructor for a medical–surgical clinical rotation for senior nursing students. Review the mission, philosophy, and clinical objectives for this rotation. Design clinical experiences for these students that will help them meet clinical objectives.
2. You are the clinical faculty for the obstetrics–pediatrics nursing course and responsible for planning clinical experiences for the students. When determining the appropriateness of the clinical experience, which criteria will you consider before assigning students to an agency?
3. You are hired as clinical faculty for a junior-level nursing clinical rotation. You will be taking your students to an acute care hospital on a medical–surgical unit designated as a Dedicated Education Unit. Create a list of faculty responsibilities that you will need to ensure are met, and schedule these responsibilities on your semester calendar.

REFERENCES

Ali, P. A., & Panther, W. (2008). Professional development and the role of mentorship. *Nursing Standard, 22*(42), 35–39.

American Association of Colleges of Nursing (AACN). (2012). Guiding principles. Retrieved from http://www.aacn.nche.edu/leading-initiatives/academic-practice-partnerships/GuidingPrinciples.pdf

American Association of Colleges of Nursing (AACN). (2016). The essential clinical resources for nursing's academic mission. Retrieved from http://www.aacn.nche.edu/education-resources/essential-clinical-resources

Beal, J. (2012). Academic-service partnerships in nursing: An integrative review. *Nursing Research and Practice, 2012*, 1–12, article ID501564.

Billings, D. M., & Halstead, J. A. (Eds.). (2016). *Teaching in nursing: A guide for faculty* (5th ed.). St. Louis, MO: WB Saunders.

Gaberson, K., & Oermann, M. (2015). *Clinical teaching strategies in nursing* (4th ed.). New York, NY: Springer.

Goode, C., Lynn, M. R., Krsek, C., & Bednash, G. D. (2009). Nurse residency programs: An essential requirement for nursing. *Nursing Economics, 27*(3), 142–147.

Institute of Medicine. (2010). *The future of nursing: Leading change, advancing health.* Washington, DC: National Academies of Health.

Moscato, S. R., Miller, J., Logsdon, K., Weinberg, S., & Chorpenning, L. (2007). Dedicated education unit: An innovative clinical partner education model. *Nursing Outlook, 55*(1), 31–37.

Shpritz, D. W., & O'Mara, A. M. (2006). Model preceptor program for student nurses. In J. P. Flynn & M. C. Stack (Eds.), *The role of the preceptor* (pp. 28–52). Boston, MA: Springer.

University Health System Consortium (UHSC) & American Association of Colleges of Nursing (AACN). (2008). Background. Retrieved from http://www.aacn.nche.edu/leading-initiatives/education-resources/NurseResidencyProgramExecSumm.pdf

University Health System Consortium (UHSC) & American Association of Colleges of Nursing (AACN). (2016). Nurse residency program. Retrieved from http://www.aacn.nche.edu/education-resources/NRPParticipants.pdf

U.S. Department of Health and Human Services. (n.d.). Health information privacy. Retrieved from http://www.hhs.gov/hipaa/index.html

CHAPTER 8

Preparation for Your Clinical Teaching Assignment

OBJECTIVES

- Identify faculty responsibilities in preparation for the beginning of a clinical teaching assignment in a healthcare agency.
- Value the importance of establishing interpersonal relationships with clinical agency personnel.
- Assess a clinical agency for appropriate learning experiences that will enhance student learning outcomes.
- Develop an orientation plan to help students with their transition to the clinical agency and their ability to achieve the expected clinical outcomes.
- Apply the nurse educator competencies in the clinical setting.

Nursing faculty responsibilities include clinical teaching. Just as you need to prepare for teaching in the classroom, so you need to prepare to teach on a clinical unit. Faculty need to make any necessary arrangements with clinical agencies and unit staff prior to the arrival of the nursing students. Once all contracts between the school of nursing and the clinical agency have been signed and you receive your clinical assignment for the semester, you and the other nursing faculty have certain responsibilities that can help ensure a smooth transition for the nursing students onto the clinical unit. This chapter will address your responsibilities when preparing for that clinical teaching assignment.

GETTING STARTED

The length and location of your clinical teaching assignment will vary depending on the nursing curriculum. Your clinical assignment commitment may be for one or two days weekly over various semester periods. The length of each clinical day will also vary depending on the program time frame. For example, you may be hired as a clinical instructor to bring students to a clinical setting one day a week for eight hours each day throughout a 15-week semester. Where you bring students for their clinical experience will depend on the course objectives. For this reason, it is important for you to be familiar with the course with which this clinical assignment is associated. You need to have a copy of the course syllabus identifying the course content as well as the clinical objectives and expected student outcomes. This information will help you plan clinical experiences for the students that help them achieve the course and clinical objectives.

You also need to understand the guidelines for clinical assignments as well as the grading criteria for these assignments. If specific rubrics are used to evaluate assignments, these rubrics need to be shared with you. Clinical faculty need to be familiar with the clinical evaluation tool and what constitutes an acceptable level of student performance at each level of the program; for example, students at the beginning of their clinical experiences may demonstrate beginning critical thinking behaviors, whereas more advanced students independently initiate critical thinking to address clinical situations.

In addition to a list of students assigned to your clinical rotation, you will need pragmatic information that will help organize semester activities, such as clinical start and end dates, due dates for clinical assignments, mid-term and final evaluations, clinical observations and off-campus activities as needed, and any scheduled school closings during the semester. Students also need to know how they can contact you in the event of an emergency. Provide them with an email address or telephone number along with the expected notification time frame.

You should also request a copy of the student handbook. In addition to finding the policies and procedures related to student progression through the nursing program, you will find policies and procedures related to students' responsibilities in the clinical setting in the handbook. The topics covered may include student attendance, management of student injury, and procedures for handling patient care errors.

If you have been hired as an adjunct clinical instructor, it is important for you to maintain open and frequent communication with the lead instructor for the course. Because clinical instructors often are not on campus at regular times, you may begin to feel disconnected from full-time faculty. Communication between full-time faculty and clinical adjuncts is crucial to maintaining quality clinical experiences for students. These open communication channels are important for sharing student progress and any issues that may arise in the clinical setting requiring immediate attention. Alternate plans for helping students improve their performance to meet clinical objectives also can be discussed.

As a member of the clinical faculty, you are responsible for ensuring students learn to deliver nursing care in a safe, knowledgeable manner. Working as a team with the lead instructor can help ensure students have safe and meaningful clinical experiences.

MEETING WITH THE CLINICAL AGENCY STAFF

As you know, clinical agencies may include acute care hospitals, long-term and rehabilitation facilities, as well as various outpatient settings. The agency where you will bring the students will, once again, depend on the program curriculum. Schools of nursing select clinical agencies that will facilitate the achievement of course objectives and student learning outcomes. For example, if students are enrolled in a community health nursing course, clinical assignments may include outpatient facilities.

Regardless of the clinical agency used for the course, nursing faculty need to work as a team with agency personnel and establish a trusting relationship with them. Establishing this trust begins with clinical faculty meeting with important nursing personnel such as the nurse manager, the nurse educator, and the agency professional and nonprofessional staff prior to the students' arrival at the agency. These meetings should be scheduled at least one month before the beginning of the clinical rotation. These initial meetings are important because they set the foundation for the development of trusting relationships between the school of nursing faculty and agency staff. These meetings will help you and the agency staff become more familiar with the roles, responsibilities, and legal obligations of all parties involved with providing learning experiences for the nursing students.

During your meetings with the nurse manager and nurse educator, you need to share the course syllabus and student schedule. This will help the nurse manager and nurse educator become familiar with the mission and philosophy of the school of nursing, course content, clinical objectives, and student learning outcomes. They will also learn the days and times of the week to expect the students on their unit. This is also the time for you to learn about any agency policies and procedures as they relate to faculty and student responsibilities assigned to the agency for the clinical learning experience. At these meetings, the nurse manager and the nurse educator may share with you any specific activities or forms that need to be completed by the students prior to their arrival on the unit. Contact phone numbers and addresses for faculty and students should also be shared with the nurse manager and nurse educator, if requested. Arrangements for parking on site and use of conference rooms and locker space may be discussed at these meetings. Likewise, any special assignments or observations that faculty may want students to experience in addition to their routine assignments may be discussed and arranged at these meetings. Any documentation required by the school of nursing and the agency at the completion of the clinical rotation may be discussed as well.

After meeting with the nurse manager and the nurse educator, faculty should also meet with the professional and nonprofessional nursing staff. This meeting helps the staff become familiar with the mission and philosophy of the school of nursing, course content, clinical objectives, and student learning outcomes. When you meet with the staff, you can share the course syllabus and student schedule. The students' clinical schedule is shared with the staff so they know the days and times to expect the students and can be prepared to engage in the students' learning experiences. More importantly, this meeting helps the staff understand their relationship with the students and their role in providing for the educational experiences of students. At these meetings you will provide staff with a review of the students' clinical expectations and the competencies they need to achieve from this clinical rotation. Staff are given the opportunity to learn their role as preceptors who help facilitate this learning. Some schools of nursing may have a preceptor orientation for staff nurses who will assume the role of preceptor in the clinical setting.

Your meeting with professional and nonprofessional staff can help build trusting relationships between you and the employees on the agency unit. Agency staff need to know you will keep them informed of students' assignments and any patient care events as they occur on the clinical unit. Staff on the unit also need to know that students are expected to keep the agency staff informed about the patient care they have delivered and any changes in the patients' condition. In addition, staff need to know faculty value their input regarding students' abilities to deliver safe nursing care that satisfy patients' priority needs. In some nursing programs, clinical faculty may also seek staff input into the students' clinical evaluation.

VISITING THE CLINICAL AGENCY

After meeting with agency staff you should arrange to visit the agency or clinical unit. The purpose of this visit is for you to assess the learning environment and determine the availability of learning opportunities that will help students meet their learning outcomes. Hosoda (2006) developed a Clinical Learning Environment Diagnostic Inventory (CLEDI) that is useful for assessing learning environments in clinical settings. Drawing from Kolb's (1984) experiential learning theory and Schon's (1983) epistemology of practice, this instrument measures five dimensions of the clinical learning environment—affective, perceptual, symbolic, behavioral, and reflective. You may want to review the CLEDI when assessing the clinical learning environment where you will be teaching nursing students.

This visit will also help you become more familiar with the roles of agency staff and how these roles enhance the daily operations of the agency or clinical unit. When you are given this opportunity to experience firsthand agency routines in the delivery of patient care, you can better prepare for the students' active engagement in the role of the professional nurse in this environment. Of course, one of the best ways for you to learn about nursing care delivery on this unit may be to spend a day "working" with the staff. Spending a day with staff may be beneficial for you if this is your first time in this clinical environment. Once you have been a clinical instructor at this agency many times, it may not be necessary for you to spend a day with the staff because you have already learned unit operations, and staff relationships have been cemented.

When you visit the clinical agency, you are there to evaluate the appropriateness of this unit in helping students meet clinical objectives and have a good learning experience. Therefore, there are a few important questions to keep in mind when you visit the agency:

- Which learning experiences are available in relation to course content, skills development, patient teaching, and interdisciplinary communication?
- What is the patient acuity level, turnover rate, and overall pace of unit operations, which may influence opportunities for student learning?
- What are nurse–patient staffing ratios, and how are they determined? Do staff seem to have the time to engage in the student learning process?
- What are the overall qualifications of the staff for the job they do? Does the unit consist of experienced practitioners, or are many staff new to their positions? Do the staff seem to be receptive to the opportunity to work with students?
- What is the layout of the physical environment? Is the unit designed so that you can easily visualize the students while they deliver care? Is the nursing work area large enough to accommodate the students; if not, is there a conference space where students can gather? How are important messages about unit operations related to patient flow communicated? Are there daily postings in the nursing work area that help staff organize unit operations?
- How is technology used in the delivery of patient care? Is the electronic medical record (EMR) used by all professional and nonprofessional staff to record patient care? Do students have access to the EMR, or is this access restricted only to faculty?
- Are there adequate resources available to administer patient care? How are patient care supplies obtained? Do students have direct access to these supplies, or do they need to be obtained only by the instructor? Which equipment is available for student use? Is this equipment state-of-the-art or outdated? Do you have a basic working knowledge of the equipment available to students?

Once you have obtained the answers to these questions and perhaps spent a day with the agency staff, you will be in a better position to plan clinical learning experiences for your students that will help them meet the clinical objectives.

GETTING TO KNOW YOUR CLINICAL STUDENTS

It is important to meet with your clinical students at the beginning of the clinical assignment. You may be able to meet with these students before the first day of the clinical experience, or this meeting may take place on the first clinical day. Faculty need to establish a time and place for this initial meeting. If this meeting will be at the agency, faculty need to provide the students with directions to the facility and information on parking regulations and fees. Depending on the length of the clinical day, students need to know about any available mealtime accommodations. In addition, they need to know about proper attire (uniforms, lab coats, street clothes), use of identification tags, and equipment needed, such as stethoscopes, penlights, scissors, and electronic devices. Students also need to know if they will have a place to safely store their valuables. You may want to consider sending this information in an email to your clinical students before you meet with them. Meeting with the students prior to the start of the clinical assignment may also be a time when you can have students complete all preliminary documentation needed by the agency before they can start the clinical rotation.

At the clinical site, your initial meeting with the students should begin by giving the students the opportunity to get to know you. Share your excitement about the clinical learning experience and your role in helping them achieve clinical objectives. From the beginning, students need to be able to trust you will create a learning environment that will help decrease their anxiety and encourage them to take an active part in their learning experiences. To do this, you may want to share with the students your feelings about your role as an educator. When conveying your beliefs about your role as an educator, you should discuss the importance of establishing collegial relationships, allowing students the freedom to learn by taking risks, and facing challenges without fear of misjudgment. Students need to know you are open to communication and encourage collaborative problem solving. They need to know the constructive criticism you may provide is being done to build their confidence and help them succeed. Students also need to know of your experience as a clinical educator and feel confident in your abilities. You may want to share with the students your experiences as a nurse and educator, your advanced education degrees, and some information about your family makeup and hobbies. Once students know your abilities as a nurse and educator and later are given the opportunity to experience your instructor role in action, they may value their clinical learning experiences and aspire to higher standards of practice. In a comparative study among nursing students, the four important qualities possessed by effective clinical instructors were professional competence, interpersonal relationship, personality characteristics, and teaching ability (Yang, Chou, & Chiang, 2005).

After you have introduced yourself to the clinical group, have each member of the group introduce himself or herself. These introductions may include the student's education, work history, family life, hobbies, reasons for choosing nursing as a career, and expectations for this clinical experience. As you begin to listen to the students' stories, you may gain an appreciation for the students' past life experiences and their future goals as members of the nursing profession. Knowledge of your students' backgrounds may help you choose learning experiences that are meaningful and directed toward their future goals.

Many times the students in your clinical group may know one another from taking previous courses together or being assigned to the same clinical group at another time in the curriculum. Regardless, this initial meeting among these group members can spark the formation of the team spirit needed to enhance this learning experience. Students may begin to feel more connected to their classmates and work together to help each other achieve the clinical objectives. In other words, learning becomes a joint effort.

Students also should be introduced to the staff on the clinical unit. This step may help contribute to the development of practice learning teams between the student and the clinical nurse. Ott and Succheralli (2015) noted this collaborative learning had a positive impact on teamwork, the students' clinical learning experiences, and their clinical confidence level as future nurses.

You may also want to review each student's academic record and previous clinical evaluations to get a sense of the student's clinical competence; however, conducting such a review may bias your evaluation of the student. Instead, nursing faculty need to use a range of clinical evaluation strategies to help strive for fairness and objectivity in their evaluations while helping to ensure consistency across faculty evaluations (Oermann et al., 2009). Your responsibility for performing clinical evaluations is discussed in Chapter 10.

ORIENTATION TO THE CLINICAL AGENCY FOR FACULTY AND STUDENTS

Although you have already met with agency staff, you may also be required to attend a formalized orientation for clinical instructors sponsored by the agency's education department. Many agencies will not let clinical instructors bring students to the facility unless the clinical instructor has attended the yearly orientation program. Usually this orientation will address those policies and procedures related to faculty/student responsibilities at the facility and use of the electronic medical record (EMR). Agencies have regulations defining who may access the EMR. Some agencies will allow only the clinical instructor to have this access, whereas others will also allow students to chart in the EMR. In either case, the appropriate people need to be given the necessary access codes, which should occur on orientation day. Faculty must attend orientation day when required by the clinical agency. Payment for your attendance at this orientation is determined by the school of nursing that hired you.

Orientation for students assigned to an agency is usually done on the first clinical day. Usually this orientation does not include students receiving a patient assignment; however, depending on the length of the clinical day, students may receive a patient assignment after the orientation is completed. Some agencies may provide the students with a basic orientation to the facility's mission and philosophy; policies and procedures related to safety, infection control, and patients' rights; and Health Insurance Portability and Accountability Act (HIPAA) regulations. If the agency does not provide this basic orientation to nursing students, you will need to do this. You will also need to provide the students with a tour of the unit and an introduction to the staff. In some cases, the nurse manager or staff designee may provide this tour of the unit. A tour of the unit should include how to operate the equipment (e.g., bed controls, call bell systems, oxygen and IV machines), medication administration protocols and equipment, charting procedures, and use of the EMR.

In an undergraduate nursing program, one fun-filled way students can be oriented to the physical environment is through a scavenger hunt that they complete on their first clinical day. This exercise will help students become more familiar with the location of equipment and supplies. Two or three students can work together to locate the items on the list. (**Box 8-1** contains a sample scavenger hunt list.) You may want to limit the time for this exercise to about one hour and then meet with the students to determine whether all items have been found. An exercise like this encourages students to work collaboratively from the beginning of the clinical rotation.

In graduate nursing programs, a scavenger hunt generally is not needed; instead, students can complete a checklist of things to do (see **Box 8-2**). Graduate students may be given a list of important activities for them to complete throughout the clinical rotation. These may include meeting with individuals from departments at the college who may impact upon the operations of the nursing program, attending specific meetings related to the role of the nurse educator, planning teaching projects that include developing and implementing teaching plans and evaluation methods, observing clinical faculty in their supervision of nursing students, and assisting clinical faculty throughout the clinical rotation.

After students have completed the scavenger hunt or reviewed their to-do list, you will need to meet with them to review the clinical objectives and the expectations for their clinical learning rotations.

DISCUSSING EXPECTATIONS FOR THE CLINICAL EXPERIENCE

After you and your clinical students have had an opportunity to get to know each other, meet agency personnel, and become oriented to the physical environment, faculty need to discuss student responsibilities during their clinical experience. When you meet with students to discuss what is expected from them, you are setting the ground rules and structure for the learning experience while giving the students opportunities to ask questions. Areas to be discussed are included in **Box 8-3**.

During this time you will want to go over the clinical objectives and the student assignments that will help students meet clinical outcomes. You need to provide students with a clinical schedule for when the clinical rotation begins and ends as well as the

Box 8-1 Scavenger Hunt for Undergraduate Nursing Programs

Working in groups of two or three, students need to find the items listed here. Identify the exact location of each item.

- Linens, washcloths, and towels
- Bandages, tape, and dressing sponges
- Soap, toothbrushes, toothpaste, mouthwash, and combs
- Wash basins
- Bed pans
- Blood pressure machine
- Thermometers
- Pulse oximeter
- Crash cart
- Intubation box
- Portable monitor
- Face masks and oxygen tanks
- IV solutions, electronic IV machines, and tubing
- Glucometers
- Feeding tubes and machines
- Gloves, gowns, and masks
- Fire extinguishers

Box 8-2 To-Do List in a Graduate Nursing Program

Listed below are a few activities you will need to complete prior to the end of this clinical rotation.

Meet with ancillary department members:
- Admissions
- Registration
- Counseling
- Health Services
- Other _____

Attend nursing department meetings:
- General department meetings
- Curriculum
- Recruitment and retention
- Program evaluation
- Other _____

(*continued*)

Box 8-2 To-Do List in a Graduate Nursing Program (*continued*)

Attend college-wide committee meetings:
- Senate
- Curriculum
- Admissions
- Other _____

Teaching project:
- Develop teaching plan
- Develop evaluation methods
- Implement teaching project
- Other _____

Clinical practicum:
- Observe clinical faculty during rotation
- Assist clinical faculty during rotation
- Supervise student(s)
- Create assignment (s) or learning experience(s)
- Counsel student(s)
- Evaluate student(s)

Box 8-3 Expectations for the Clinical Experience

1. Review clinical objectives.
2. Review clinical schedule, dates, and times, including lateness/absenteeism policy.
3. Discuss the dress code.
4. Explain assignments and due dates.
5. Discuss role behaviors and relationships with agency staff.
6. Discuss scope of practice, delivery of care limitations as students, and seeking guidance from faculty and staff.
7. Discuss communication with faculty and agency staff.
8. Describe the organization of nursing care using the nursing process.
9. Review maintaining alertness to safety issues.

dates when these clinical assignments are to be completed. The schedule for the clinical rotation also needs to include a review of the policies for lateness, absenteeism, and any college cancellation of classes. You may also want to review the clinical dress code at this time.

You will also want to review with students the expectations for their professional role behaviors during the clinical rotation. In an undergraduate nursing program, students' clinical experiences will be managed collaboratively with oversight from their faculty or clinical preceptors. In graduate nursing programs, students who are registered nurses may function more autonomously under the guidance of nursing program faculty and clinical practitioners at the agency. In either learning situation, students are accountable for their professional actions in the delivery of patient care. They are expected to function as knowledgeable, honest, and trustworthy students who safely apply the skills they learned in the classroom. Students are also expected to maintain open communications with faculty and agency staff.

Students are required to deliver nursing care to their assigned patients within their scope of practice and agency policies and procedures. They are expected to recognize their own limitations, ask questions, and seek assistance when needed. Any change in the patient's condition needs to be reported to the faculty and staff promptly, not at the end of the day. Students need to demonstrate initiative in the planning of their nursing care and not expect faculty or staff to continuously direct the plan for patient care. Instead, students need to work collaboratively with agency staff to satisfy patient care needs. Students also are expected to give faculty and appropriate agency staff an end-of-shift report about the nursing care given to their assigned patients as well as the status of their patients at the end of the day.

Students have difficulty organizing their responsibilities when delivering patient care. To help students organize their nursing care, you may want to review with them the steps in the nursing process and how these steps (assess, plan, implement, and evaluate) are implemented in the clinical setting. Be specific about when and how students are to assess their patients. Encourage each student to obtain the patient's vital signs and perform a head-to-toe patient assessment at the beginning of the clinical day. Remind students of the need to reassess vital signs as per the agency policy and when there is a change in the patient's condition. Also point out to students the need to assess the treatments the patient is receiving, such as oxygen therapy, IV fluids, enteral feedings, and urinary drainage systems.

Once students have assessed their patients and the treatments they are receiving, they should follow the next step of the nursing process and begin planning for the delivery of nursing care to their assigned patients. This planning process needs to include a review of the physician's orders. Reviewing the physician's orders will help the students know when medications are to be administered, when laboratory or diagnostic tests are to be done, the patient's diet, the patient's activity level, and any other special nursing care needs each patient may have. Once students are aware of their patients' nursing care needs, they can begin to implement this nursing care.

When implementing nursing care, students are expected to prioritize their delivery of care. The ability to prioritize nursing care can be a difficult task; some students are more skilled at this task than others. Helping students prioritize nursing care is an important role for faculty or the preceptor. After students have assessed their patients and know the plans of care, you may want to encourage students to discuss with you their plan for patient care delivery. Having this discussion with the students may help them think critically about how to prioritize patient care. For example, suppose the patient has medications scheduled for 10 in the morning and a dressing change to be done once a shift. Your discussion with the student may address the question, "What do you do first, and why?" Students' responses to this question may help you evaluate their ability to set priorities for patient care while identifying those students who are weaker in this area and need more assistance from you. Students are fully responsible for the care they deliver to their assigned patients; when the delivery of this care involves a nursing skill they do not feel competent to perform, students need to know they are expected to come to the faculty or preceptor for help.

Students also need to know they are expected to evaluate the delivery of their patient care throughout the entire time they are assigned to the patients. Any complaints or changes in patients' condition need to be reassessed and reported immediately to the faculty or preceptor. When evaluating the outcomes of their nursing care on their patients, students are expected to propose revisions in their care that may be beneficial to their patients. Students must understand that any proposed revisions in care need to be discussed with the faculty or preceptor before the changes are implemented.

Finally, the need to maintain safety when administering nursing care needs to be strongly emphasized with students. Students need to know they are expected to demonstrate the ability to safely perform the nursing skills taught to them in the laboratory by adhering to procedures and safety criteria. They should not independently perform any nursing skills that were not taught to them in the laboratory or skills they lack the confidence to perform. Instead, they need to seek out the assistance of the faculty or preceptor when these situations arise. Remind students that they are responsible for the patient care they administer and will be held accountable for incidents that may occur because they did not seek the appropriate guidance when needed. Tell students that faculty and preceptors will assign patients who give students the opportunity to learn from experience. Students need to know that exposure to these challenging patients will test the limits of their ability and require them to identify their own limitations. You will need to reassure students that faculty and preceptors are available to answer their questions and help them maintain patient safety.

SATISFYING NURSE EDUCATOR COMPETENCIES IN THE CLINICAL SETTING

Chapter 1 presented the National League for Nursing (NLN) core competencies for nurse educators. Let us now examine how these core competencies can be applied by faculty in the clinical setting.

Competency 1: Facilitate Learning

To facilitate learning in the clinical setting you need to be knowledgeable about the content students have learned in the classroom and laboratory for the clinical course level you are teaching, as well as the clinical objectives and the student outcomes expected at the end of this clinical experience. The teaching strategies you use should be varied, be grounded in educational theory, and consider differences in learner styles and cultural influences. The clinical experiences you plan for students should give them opportunities to apply what they have learned in the classroom and laboratory settings. These experiences may progress by first assigning patients who require basic skills, such as bathing, ambulating, turning, and positioning, and then gradually assigning patients requiring more complex skills, such as suctioning, dressing changes, and medication administration. When assigning patients to the students, you may want to consider how often they have been in the clinical setting as students. Students are more anxious when they first begin caring for patients, but with experience they should become more comfortable with their role and responsibilities. As students become more comfortable with their role in the clinical setting, faculty should assign patients who have more challenging healthcare needs. This will allow students to gain more of the knowledge and skills required as a registered nurse.

As students administer nursing care to their assigned patients, you may want to ask them questions about the care they are giving and the patients' responses to this treatment. By doing this, faculty may create opportunities for students to develop their critical thinking and critical reasoning skills (Hoffman, 2008). At times, students may feel intimidated with your line of questioning, but if you have clearly explained from the beginning your purpose for asking questions, students may welcome these questions more readily.

Students' perceptions of you in the clinical setting can influence learning. Lovecchio and colleagues (2015) noted students' satisfaction with clinical learning improved when faculty made clear assignments, provided specific instructions, maintained organization, and provided individualized attention. Therefore, it is important for you to develop relationships with your students that demonstrate personal attributes such as respect for them as learners, confidence in their ability to succeed, patience with them when they are struggling, and encouragement to help them obtain higher standards of practice. Finally, you should be that role model they may want to emulate one day as nurses.

Competency 2: Facilitate Learner Development and Socialization

An important responsibility for you as clinical faculty is to help students develop confidence in their ability to deliver nursing care and to prepare them to function as beginning practitioners in the healthcare environment. One way to do this is to provide a learning environment that fosters cognitive, psychomotor, and affective learning. To develop these abilities in students you need to help them relate the nursing knowledge learned in the classroom to the delivery of care in the clinical setting. For example, if patients have respiratory problems, the student needs to understand the physiological and psychological changes that can happen to these patients and provide the appropriate nursing care that addresses these changes. Remember, facilitating learner development does not mean you, as an instructor, take on the teaching role of *showing* students how to care for their patients' specific needs. Instead, it means you need to *step back* in your teaching role and allow students to take control of their learning by independently attending to patients' needs while you are present to assist them if requested. Faculty cannot continue to show students how to deliver safe nursing care—faculty need to learn to let go. This may help students develop self-confidence in their ability to deliver safe nursing care. However, if students are struggling to deliver safe nursing care, you may intercede by showing them the correct way to deliver care.

As faculty, it is also your role to help students engage in self-reflection by identifying their own strengths and weakness. At times, attempting to do this may be uncomfortable for beginning nurse educators who feel a lack of confidence in their own new role. After you have had time to identify your own strengths and weakness as an educator, you will begin to feel more comfortable discussing this topic with your students. When evaluating students, providing constructive feedback may also help with student development. When you provide constructive feedback, it needs to be precise and specific, identifying the specific areas of knowledge that are lacking, techniques that need improvement, and problems in critical thinking and clinical judgments (Gaberson & Oermann, 2010). However, a word of caution is needed about giving constructive feedback. Some students may erroneously personalize what you have to say about their nursing care and subsequently become very defensive about their actions. It is your responsibility to guide students through a self-reflection process that can help the students understand their own limitations, identify their errors, and establish ways to improve their practice (Bonnel, 2008). This will help students understand why you are providing this constructive feedback.

Faculty also need to create an environment that focuses on the socialization of students to their future roles as registered nurses. To help with this socialization, faculty need to take into consideration the cultural diversity of the students and how students' cultural backgrounds may influence their perceptions of how health care is delivered. Faculty also need to familiarize students with the various cultural beliefs that may impact their delivery of nursing care. Students need to learn the importance of integrating cultural awareness, cultural sensitivity, and cultural competence into their nursing care (Kleiman, Frederickson, & Lundy, 2004). For example, many cultures believe it to be the responsibility of the family to care for their elderly at home when they can no longer care for themselves, whereas in the United States extended long-term care and hospice services are available for the elderly when they can no longer care for themselves.

Another important responsibility of the nurse educator is to provide advisement and counseling to students when the need arises. It is usually the clinical faculty who first identify when students are not adjusting well to their role as future nurses. Many times students enter a nursing program without a clear understanding of the role of the professional nurse in the delivery of health care. As students engage in their clinical experiences, they may begin to question whether this is a profession they want to enter. When students begin to second-guess their goal of becoming a nurse, this may begin to manifest itself in the quality of their nursing care. When faculty first identify this behavior in their students, they need to provide effective advisement and counseling by encouraging students to speak with career counselors. Some students are encouraged by their families to become nurses, and unfortunately later realize this is not the profession for them. Other students may have personal family issues that prevent them from dedicating time to their studies. Faculty may need to encourage these students to speak with academic counselors.

Competency 3: Use Assessment and Evaluation Strategies

Clinical faculty need to be able to use a variety of strategies to assess and evaluate students' abilities to achieve the expected learner outcomes. Using a variety of methods, faculty are able to measure students' abilities to deliver safe nursing care in the cognitive, psychomotor, and affective domains. Faculty also use these assessment and evaluation data to enhance the teaching/learning process. Faculty need to be aware of the different evaluation methods used in the clinical setting so they will be able to determine students' progression toward achieving the desired clinical outcomes. Throughout the clinical experience, faculty need to provide timely, constructive, and thoughtful feedback to students that will help them achieve the expected outcomes for this clinical experience. These assessment and evaluation strategies will be presented in more depth in Chapter 10.

Competency 4: Participate in Curriculum Design and Evaluation of Program Outcomes

If you are full-time faculty in a nursing program, participation in curriculum development and program evaluation are a major part of your responsibilities as a nurse educator. Clinical faculty, in contrast, may not have direct, hands-on involvement with these responsibilities because they have been hired to teach only in the clinical component of the program. However, that is not to say your input into curriculum development and program evaluation cannot be of value. Nurses hired as clinical faculty usually have full-time employment in a clinical agency. This full-time employment keeps them up-to-date on current healthcare delivery trends and the roles and responsibilities of nurses in a dynamic, changing healthcare environment. This knowledge and experience can contribute to the development of much-needed learner competencies within the nursing curriculum. Therefore, as a member of the clinical faculty you may want to collaborate with full-time faculty throughout the process of curriculum revision so the identified learner needs address current societal and healthcare trends.

Competency 5: Function as Change Agent and Leader

As a nurse educator with clinical teaching responsibilities, you function as a change agent and leader by participating in interdisciplinary efforts to address healthcare and educational needs. You do this by preparing the future nursing force with the skills and knowledge needed to practice in the current healthcare environment. This takes collegial efforts between the school of nursing and the healthcare agency to create and maintain community and clinical partnerships that support educational goals. Many times advisory boards, made up of faculty and agency administrators, are created to link practice needs with the educational goals of the nursing program. Nurse educators, including clinical instructors, need to be active members of these advisory boards. Usually these advisory boards will meet once or twice a year during the fall and/or spring semesters. The boards are made up of administrators from the nursing program and clinical agency, faculty from the school of nursing, and mid-level administrators and select nursing staff from the clinical agency.

Clinical educators can also be change agents for the school of nursing by keeping the school aware of how the role of the nurse is changing in various healthcare settings. Clinical faculty need to be present at the school of nursing department meetings. At these meetings, clinical faculty may provide the leadership needed to promote innovative and creative practices that can be integrated into the nursing curriculum. Recognizing and implementing this input from clinical faculty may identify strategies for change within schools of nursing.

Competency 6: Pursue Continuous Quality Improvement in the Nurse Educator Role

Nurse educators in the clinical setting need to strive for quality improvement among their students. To do this means expecting high standards of practice from your students. When students are not meeting those expected standards of practice, it becomes your responsibility to help them do so by providing them with professional development opportunities to increase their effectiveness. This begins by providing them with feedback describing their strengths and weaknesses and developing a plan of action to help them improve. This plan of action needs to be established early in the clinical rotation so students are aware of the resources available and have time to improve upon those expected standards. This plan of action will be discussed further in Chapter 10.

As a nurse educator, it is your responsibility to maintain a commitment to lifelong learning. For some this may mean pursuing additional formal degrees in higher education, receiving certification as a Certified Nurse Educator (CNE), or attending continuing education programs in teaching and learning.

Competency 7: Engage in Scholarship

Nurse educators need to introduce their students to the importance of nursing scholarship. Students need to know that the expected standards of nursing practice are grounded in evidence-based practices. To achieve this in the clinical setting, faculty may want to assign a project to a group of students that explores the research literature about a specific nursing skill or patient teaching project. This type of assignment introduces students to the concept of evidence-based practice and may foster a spirit of inquiry into acceptable standards of nursing care. Students can also be assigned to develop and implement patient teaching projects grounded in evidence-based research.

Competency 8: Function Within the Educational Environment

Although this competency outlines the professional activities of a nurse educator, you can begin to promote this competency in your nursing students by encouraging them to become members of the student nurses association. As members of their professional organizations, students can learn early in their career the importance of developing networks with other nursing professionals. These networks help establish professional and collegial relationships that may one day help them find jobs to meet their professional goals. Students' continued membership in professional organizations after graduation also may help them assume leadership roles as advocates for the nursing profession in the political arena.

SUMMARY

This chapter has presented information about what faculty need to know to prepare for their clinical teaching assignments. To be well prepared for their clinical teaching assignments and to facilitate clinical learning experiences for the students, faculty need to be familiar with the information contained in the course syllabus, the course and clinical objectives, and the clinical schedule. To enhance relationships between the school of nursing and clinical agencies, faculty also need to meet with all levels of agency personnel who may be directly involved with the students' learning experiences. Faculty need to review with agency personnel the course syllabus, the course and clinical objectives, and the time schedule when students will be present at the agency. Once you have attended to all these preliminary obligations, you will be ready to bring students to the clinical agency for their learning experiences.

CASE STUDY

You were hired as clinical faculty in a nursing program at a nearby university. This is your first experience in this role. Your clinical teaching assignment is at a 500-bed acute care hospital on a medical–surgical unit. You have 10 students in this clinical rotation who are sophomores in the nursing program.

1. Develop a list of responsibilities you will need to accomplish before bringing students to this clinical facility.
2. Which questions do you want to ask about this clinical learning environment to determine whether this clinical unit will provide the needed clinical learning experiences to satisfy student learning outcomes?
3. Develop an orientation to help students with their transition to the clinical agency and their ability to achieve the expected clinical outcomes. You will provide orientation on the first eight-hour clinical day. Create an orientation schedule, and be sure to include the following:
   - Establishing relationships among you, the staff, and the students
   - Clinical unit policies and procedures relevant to nursing students
   - The physical unit and the location of supplies and equipment
   - Student responsibilities during the clinical experience

REFERENCES

Bonnel, W. (2008). Improving feedback to students in online courses. *Nursing Education Perspectives, 29,* 290–294.

Gaberson, K. B., & Oermann, M. H. (2010). *Clinical teaching strategies in nursing* (3rd ed.). New York, NY: Springer.

Hoffman, J. (2008). Teaching strategies to facilitate nursing students' critical thinking. *Annual Review of Nursing Education, 6,* 225–236.

Hosoda, Y. (2006). Development and testing of a Clinical Learning Environment Diagnostic Inventory for baccalaureate nursing students. *Journal of Advanced Nursing, 56*(5), 480–490.

Kolb, D. A. (1984). *Experiential learning: Experience as the source of learning and development.* Upper Saddle River, NJ: Prentice Hall.

Lovecchio, C., DiMattio, M. J. K., & Hudacek, S. (2015). Predictors of undergraduate nursing student satisfaction with clinical learning environment: A secondary analysis. *Nursing Education Perspectives, 36*(4), 252–254.

Oermann, M. H., Yarbrough, S. S., Ard, N., Saewert, K. J., & Charasika, M. (2009). Clinical evaluation and grading practices in schools of nursing: National survey findings part II. *Nursing Education Perspectives, 30,* 274–279.

Ott, L. K., & Succheralli, L. (2015). Use of student clinical dyads as a teaching strategy to facilitate learning. *Journal of Nursing Education, 54*(3), 169–172.

Schon, D. A. (1983). *The reflective practitioner: How professionals think in action.* New York, NY: Basic Books.

Yang, F., Chou, S., & Chiang, H. (2005). Student perceptions of effective and ineffective clinical instructors. *Journal of Nursing Education, 44,* 187–192.

CHAPTER 9

Clinical Teaching

OBJECTIVES

- Explain how the theory of experiential learning can be applied in the clinical setting.
- Understand how the IOM/QSEN competencies impact your role as clinical faculty.
- Create clinical activities to address patient care needs and the experiential learning needs of students.
- Organize learning experiences, such as clinical observations, clinical conferences, and reflective journals, that contribute to students' critical thinking, clinical reasoning, and self-reflection.
- Create written assignments to evaluate students' application of the nursing process in various healthcare settings.
- Design integrated learning activities that address the *Essentials of Baccalaureate Education for Professional Nursing Practice*.

Teaching in the clinical environment is different from the teaching done by faculty in the classroom. There are no lesson plans to be followed, students are not sitting at desks taking notes, and there are no audiovisuals displayed to enhance lectures or discussions. Instead, the passive format of classroom learning becomes active learning as students take on the clinical practice component of the curriculum. In the clinical setting students have the opportunity to experience classroom learning in action. This clinical practice exposes students to information not conveyed by a textbook or lecture. In the clinical setting it is the role of faculty to facilitate this learning by providing the appropriate clinical learning activities. These clinical learning activities provide real-life situations that help students transfer classroom knowledge to practical clinical situations. This chapter will guide you in your development as a clinical faculty member capable of providing meaningful learning experiences that help students achieve successful clinical outcomes.

EXPERIENTIAL LEARNING: THE CORE OF CLINICAL TEACHING

When students go to clinical agencies they are provided with opportunities to apply their classroom knowledge, develop those nursing skills needed to care for various patient populations, learn to problem solve, and enhance their nursing judgment. These clinical rotations form the core component of experiential learning. When faculty are assigned clinical teaching, it is important for them to have some background in experiential learning because this knowledge may help them understand why faculty are encouraged to use a variety of teaching strategies to help students learn in the clinical setting.

Simply defined, experiential learning means learning from experience or learning by doing. Dewey (1938) believed that "all genuine education comes about through experience" (p. 35). He viewed experiential learning as a conscious, dialectical, problem-solving process that integrates personal experiences, concepts, observations, and actions. The interpretation of experiential learning means becoming aware of a problem, getting ideas to solve the problem, trying out a response, experiencing the consequences, and either confirming or modifying previous actions or conceptions. This interpretation of experiential learning is similar to the nursing process. When students are given the experience of caring for patients in the clinical setting, they are taught to implement the nursing process; that is, they are expected to assess their patients, plan care around patients' needs or problems, implement solutions to satisfy the needs or problems, and finally evaluate the patients' outcomes by confirming or modifying the plan of care.

Experiential learning can also be understood in terms of the effects or outcomes it has upon the learner. When our nursing students learn from experience, the expectation is for changes to occur in their behavior, knowledge, and attitudes regarding their responsibilities as future nurses. Cell (1984) references these changes by defining experiential learning as a change in what we do and how we see things. Drawing from the work of Gregory Bateson, Cell identifies four different levels of change in learners who learn from experience: a change in our behavior without changing our interpretation of the situation; a change in how we interpret the situation, our behavior, and the way we see ourselves; a change in our previous interpretations after using reflection to correct any distortions; and finally a modification of our original, underlying interpretation of a situation.

Jarvis (1987) explains how environmental context can influence a person's ability to learn from experience. He describes how people bring their cognition, emotions, physical abilities, and self-concept to the learning situation and utilize them to understand and determine how they may act. Because these personal biographies are rooted in social constructs, people will respond differently to social situations. Some may be discouraged from taking action because they are concerned about the consequences should they deviate from the expected behaviors. Jarvis concludes that "how people learn from experience and what they learn must be related to both the situation and their own biography" (p. 61). Therefore, learners' self-concepts can affect the way they interact with and respond to the learning situation. When learners have negative feelings about themselves or the situation, their understanding of the situation may be distorted and inhibit learning. Conversely, positive feelings about oneself may provide the impetus to undertake challenges, which then become learning opportunities. Because a person's emotions and self-concept may affect the learning process, it is important for faculty to develop relationships with their students that promote a positive learning environment.

For learning from experience to occur, Schon (1983) believes that professionals need to reflect upon the experience. This reflection includes the ability to step back and think about the action after it is over. Schon refers to this as both reflecting in action and reflecting on the action. This reflective thought is the antithesis of rote learning and memorization. It allows learners to construct new interpretations of the situation that may produce new techniques and knowledge. This process of using reflection to learn is similar to the process of critical thinking and clinical reasoning we read about in the nursing literature.

According to Dewey (1933), learning from experience can proceed in two different ways. The first way is through trial and error exploration without the use of reflection; the other, more effective way is through the use of *reflective activity*. Referring to reflection, Dewey wrote, "To reflect is to look back over what has been done so as to extract the net meanings which are the capital stock for intelligent dealings with further experiences. It is the heart of intellectual organization and discipline of the mind" (p. 16). Dewey believed reflection can help people find meaning in their experiences and add changed conceptual perspectives and personal growth as learner outcomes.

In summary, learning from experience can be understood as learning by doing that proceeds along a continuum from the development of skills and knowledge to alterations in meaning perspectives. However, not all experiences are learning situations. Experiential learning is influenced by a person's background and social situation and prompted by a disjuncture between these two elements. If students engage in learning from experience by using nonreflective, habitual, preconscious knowledge to satisfy the learning need of their present situation, this may result in repetitive behavior that does not necessarily contribute to their learning. In contrast, if students realize the skills and knowledge they have do not satisfy the needs of their present situation, they may contribute to their learning experience by using reflection. For this reason, when faculty develop student–patient assignments they need to expose students to a variety of learning experiences that expand on student competencies. Challenging students to expand on their present competencies encourages them to reflect on their repertoire of abilities and seek additional knowledge to help them develop the expected competencies. When students have the opportunity to reflect on their abilities and take action, learning from experience takes place. Conversely, when students are assigned patients with needs similar to past assignments, students repeat past behaviors and limit their ability to learn from experience.

ACHIEVING CORE COMPETENCIES THROUGH EXPERIENTIAL LEARNING

Nursing school programs provide clinical practicums as a component of the curriculum to help students achieve core competencies through experiences involving the delivery of nursing care. Students' experiences in these clinical practicums facilitate learning (Daley, 2001). When students are brought to the clinical setting, this is the time for you provide them with the opportunities to apply the knowledge they have learned in the classroom or laboratory to real-life patient care situations. Clinical teaching gives nursing students the chance to learn from their experiences with patient care. Therefore, as a faculty member you need to choose those patient care experiences that provide students with the best opportunities to learn the knowledge, skills, and abilities they need as beginning professional practitioners.

The Quality and Safety Education for Nurses (QSEN) project, funded by the Robert Wood Johnson Foundation, addressed the challenges faced by nursing school faculty in preparing nurses with the competencies necessary to improve quality and safety in the healthcare environment. This project resulted in the identification of six competencies that are appropriate learning outcomes for students who plan to begin basic practice as registered nurses. The QSEN faculty adapted the Institute of Medicine (IOM) competency definitions and developed the knowledge, skills, and abilities (KSAs) needed by competent nursing students who graduate from prelicensure nursing programs (Cronenwett et al., 2007). These IOM/QSEN competencies and their definitions appear in **Table 9-1**. Although it has been difficult for healthcare systems to fully implement these six competencies (Watcher, 2010), clinical nursing faculty need to continue to focus our clinical teaching around these six competencies to help ensure our students are prepared with the KSAs needed to improve the quality and safety of their nursing care delivery.

Faculty are encouraged to visit the QSEN website (www.qsen.org) to learn more about the strategies for teaching that encourage the development of the QSEN competencies in the classroom and clinical settings. This website may also provide you with ideas on evaluation methods to determine if students have achieved the knowledge,

TABLE 9-1 IOM Competencies and Definitions

Competency	Definition
Patient-Centered Care	Recognize the patient/designee as the source of control and full partner in providing compassionate and coordinated care based on respect for the patient's preferences, values, and needs.
Teamwork and Collaboration	Function effectively, within nursing and interprofessional teams, fostering open communication, mutual respect, and shared decision making to achieve quality patient care.
Evidence-Based Practice (EBP)	Integrate best current evidence with clinical expertise and patient/family preferences and values for delivery of optimal health care.
Quality Improvement (QI)	Use data to monitor the outcome of care processes and use improvement methods to design and test changes to continuously improve the quality and safety of healthcare systems.
Safety	Minimize the risk of harm to patients and providers through both system effectiveness and individual performance.
Informatics	Use information and technology to communicate, manage knowledge, mitigate error, and support decision making.

Data from Cronenwett, L., Sherwood, G., Barnsteiner, J., Disch, J., Johnson, J., Mitchell, P., . . . Warren, J. (2007). Quality and safety education for nurses. *Nursing Outlook, 55*, 122–131.

skills, and abilities they will need as beginning practitioners to help ensure the quality and safety necessary to continuously improve our healthcare systems.

CLINICAL LEARNING ASSIGNMENTS AND ACTIVITIES

When faculty begin to think about planning clinical learning activities, they need to keep in mind the clinical objectives and learner needs. In addition to being familiar with the course content found in the syllabus, you need to review the clinical objectives for the level of nursing students you have at the clinical agency. The clinical objectives help you determine the competencies your students need to achieve by the completion of their clinical rotation. The core competencies or outcomes are defined in the clinical objectives and guide the selection of learning activities. Therefore, the clinical objectives should serve as your guide for planning clinical learning assignments and activities.

When planning clinical learning assignments and activities to meet the expected competencies or outcomes, learner characteristics also need to be taken into consideration by faculty (Gaberson & Oermann, 2010). Full-time faculty who teach in the classroom and clinical setting have frequent contact with students and often know about their students' personal and professional responsibilities. Clinical faculty who are in contact with their students only in the clinical setting may not have the opportunity to know their students as well. For this reason it is important for clinical faculty to maintain open communication with the full-time faculty assigned to the course. This close contact with full-time faculty will help you keep abreast of students' progression in the curriculum. Faculty can share with you information about students' course grades and behavior in the classroom and laboratory. In addition, full-time faculty may be able to share information about other responsibilities students may have related to family and work that may interfere with their learning situations. These individual differences among your students need to be taken into consideration when planning learning activities.

Remember, faculty are available to address any questions you may have as your clinical practicum gets under way. You need to keep faculty aware of how your clinical practicum is progressing by telling them about any issues or concerns related to student performances that may emerge during the clinical rotation. As a new member of the clinical faculty, you should not hesitate to contact the full-time faculty with your questions; they are experienced educators who have probably faced similar situations and may have the best advice on how to handle the situation.

This section presents the various clinical learning assignments and activities faculty can select to help students learn the knowledge, skills, and abilities they need to successfully meet the core competencies defined in the clinical objectives. Most of these learning activities are designed to enhance critical thinking and clinical reasoning among nursing students.

Selecting Patients for Student Assignments

Before you begin to select patients for student assignments you need to consider where the students are in the nursing curriculum and what they have been learning in the classroom. Ask yourself, "Are these students beginners in the curriculum or are they at the completion of the curriculum?" The answer to this question will help you develop the student–patient assignment based on the complexity of the patient's nursing care needs and the student's knowledge. Another question you need to ask yourself when selecting a patient to assign to a student is, "How will this patient assignment help the student learn to develop the knowledge, skills, and abilities necessary for basic practice as a registered nurse who delivers safe nursing care?" When selecting these patients, you want to give your students the best opportunities to learn from their experiences. With this in mind, you may want to choose patients with complex needs who will require nursing care from a competent student. However, keeping learner characteristics in mind, you know that not all students learn at the same pace. The assignments you choose should build on students' previous knowledge and skills. To do this, you may want to ask your students which skills they have performed in other clinical rotations. Perhaps students with limited knowledge and skills need to be assigned patients with less complex needs in an effort to build their self-esteem and enable them to face more complex assignments in the future.

Faculty often wonder how many patients should be assigned to one student at any given time. This will depend on students' prior experiences in clinical practicums, the courses they have completed in the nursing program, and the complexity of patients' nursing care needs. Having more successful learning experiences in the classroom and clinical rotation should prepare students to care for more than one patient prior to graduation. As a faculty member, it should be your goal to help students learn to organize and prioritize nursing care so they may be able to care for a group of patients at the completion of the nursing program. However, you need to remember that quality is more important than quantity when assigning student–patient ratios. As Gaberson and Oermann (2010) point out, "A 2-hour activity that results in critical skill learning is far more valuable than an 8-hour activity that merely promotes repetition of skills and habit learning" (p. 13).

Once you have decided on the student–patient assignment, you need to share this assignment with the nurses on the unit, letting them know the nursing care that students will be administering. This assignment should be posted on the nursing unit for all staff to review as needed. (See an example in **Table 9-2**.) When posting this

TABLE 9-2 Nursing Student Assignment Schedule		
FACULTY: **DATE:** **TIME:** **UNIT:**		
Student Names	**Patient Assignment (Room # and Initials)**	**Nursing Care Needs/ Notes**

assignment, be sure to follow Health Insurance Portability and Accountability Act (HIPAA) regulations and maintain patient confidentiality. You should not list patients' names on the assignment form; list only room numbers and patient initials. After the nursing staff know the students assigned to their patients, they will expect the students to come to them at the beginning of the shift to receive a report on their patient.

Once all students have received reports about their patients, faculty need to direct students to begin implementing the steps in the nursing process. First, students should be expected to go into the patient's room and assess the patient by doing a physical head-to-toe examination including vital signs and checking for treatments in progress for this patient, such as IVs, enteral feedings, or oxygen therapy; checking for the presence of any tubes (e.g., Foley catheter or nasogastric or PEG feedings); and looking for any dressings or wounds that require nursing care. Once students have completed their assessment of the patient and the treatments the patient is receiving, they then begin to plan their nursing care by reviewing all physician orders. Faculty need to emphasize with students the importance of knowing physician orders at the beginning of the clinical day. Stress to students the importance of understanding the physician's orders and asking any questions if they do not understand the orders or know how to implement the skills required. Faculty should instruct students to seek assistance with skills they do not feel competent to implement.

The assignment of faculty to students in clinical settings is usually defined by the state's boards of nursing. In most states the ratio for this assignment is no more than 1 faculty member to 10 students (1:10). During a clinical rotation it is not uncommon to have 1 faculty member responsible for overseeing the nursing care of 10 students. This is a challenging responsibility for faculty, who need to provide learning situations for their students while ensuring students deliver safe nursing care to their assigned patients. In these situations, faculty need to be aware of the patients' status from the beginning of the clinical day and the students' plans for delivering care throughout the day. Here are some helpful hints.

Once students have received the report from the primary nurse and assessed their patients, have the students come to you with a report indicating their assessment findings, including vital signs and their plan for delivering nursing care. By having students provide you with this information at the beginning of the clinical day, you are able to determine if the patients are in stable condition and what treatments each student needs to deliver. You will also be able to identify which students may require your assistance due to the complexity of the patient's needs.

When students come to you with their initial report on their patients, you may also use this time to engage in a question and answer dialogue that may help identify whether your students have the knowledge, skills, and abilities to deliver nursing care safely. For example, questions addressed in the dialogue may include:

- Given this patient's vital signs and physical assessment, what is the condition of this patient? How did you come to this conclusion about the patient's condition? Given your physical assessment findings, what will you do next?
- Based on the patient report you received and the physician's orders, what are this patient's nursing care needs? What are the priority needs, and how will you organize your delivery of these needs?

Once you and the student have completed this dialogue and you have determined the student is able to deliver safe nursing care, the student is directed to proceed with care. However, if the student's responses demonstrate a limitation in his or her knowledge, skills, and abilities to deliver safe nursing care, you need to assist the student to critically think through the meanings of the assessment findings and plan of care so the student can arrive at alternative decisions and actions to ensure quality. If students express limitations in their ability to perform any procedures outlined in the physician's orders, you need to tell the students to seek your help before implementing the procedure.

Students should also be expected to keep you and the primary nurse informed about their patients' conditions. Any changes in patients' conditions need to be reported to you immediately as well as to the primary nurse. When students leave the unit for an extended period of time, such as when going to lunch or at the end of their clinical day, students should reassess their patients, including vital signs, and give updated patient reports to you and the primary nurse before they leave. Students also should be expected to document the care delivered to their patients according to agency policy. You need to review this documentation to ensure students are documenting according to the criteria taught in the classroom.

Student–Patient Ratios

Given the number of students assigned to the clinical group, faculty must decide how to set the student–patient ratio. If preceptors are used for students' clinical learning experiences, a preceptor to student–patient ratio is designed. In either case, there are several models to consider.

The traditional form of **one student to one patient** is an option. With this model, one student is responsible for meeting the comprehensive needs of one patient. The student works alone to implement the steps in the nursing process; that is, the student assesses, plans, implements, and evaluates the nursing care delivered to this patient. Faculty oversee the delivery of this care and begin to evaluate the student's capability to administer safe nursing care. This 1:1 student–patient ratio gives faculty the opportunity to become familiar with students' strengths and weaknesses. Faculty learn earlier in the clinical rotation which students are more knowledgeable and skillful and which will require more help. Faculty use anecdotal notes to help them document student progress in meeting clinical objectives and later to prepare students' final clinical evaluations. The use of anecdotal notes will be discussed further in Chapter 10.

Multiple students to one patient is another ratio option that can be chosen when patient needs are complex and will require the nursing care of more than one student. Each student takes on certain responsibilities for patient care while working as a team to meet clinical objectives. This type of assignment may help reduce student anxiety, promote collaborative learning, and help faculty identify the skill levels of the team members.

Group assignment to a specific patient population is a third option when teamwork and collaboration are the clinical objective and core competency that faculty want students to achieve. This type of ratio works best in community settings. A group of students is assigned to a specific population of patients in an outpatient clinic, and this group works together to plan clinical activities to meet the healthcare needs of this patient population. For example, a group of students might be assigned a clinical day at an adult daycare center. If faculty decide to use this student–patient ratio, they need to have specific objectives defined for this group of students before they begin to plan for this clinical activity. Faculty also need to review and approve the students' plans for this clinical activity before students are allowed to go to the outpatient facility.

Observation

Observation is another learning strategy that may be assigned to students in various clinical settings. Observational experiences can have many purposes. Observation can help students collect data about patient care delivery systems and how these systems function to maintain patient safety. Observing how practitioners identify and solve problems can help students develop abilities in clinical reasoning and decision making. The overall purpose of these clinical observations should be to promote students' understanding of nursing care delivery systems; develop higher-level thinking skills; and examine their own feelings, beliefs, and values about patient care in this specific clinical area.

Although not a primary reason for sending students to an observation, faculty workload in the clinical setting can be reduced. This can be an advantage to both faculty and students because reducing the faculty–student ratio in clinical assignments allows faculty to spend more time facilitating the learning needs of each student. When preparing students for a clinical observation, it is not enough to just send each student off to a specific clinical experience. Faculty need to have specific observational guidelines that direct students to important data they need to collect during the observation. Students need to be prepared to evaluate the observation and what they have learned from this experience. Students should be expected to share their learning experiences with the other students in a debriefing activity during clinical postconferences. When developing an observational guide, remember to keep in mind the clinical objectives and the student's level in the nursing program (**Box 9-1**).

Clinical Conferences

Conferences in clinical settings are group learning activities that can provide meaningful learning experiences for students and help bridge the gap between theory and practice. Clinical conferences are also a time when faculty can facilitate critical thinking and decision making among their students (Stokes & Kost, 2009).

Traditional clinical conferences are small group discussions that precede (preclinical conference) and follow (postconference) the students' clinical days. Preclinical conferences are a time for students to share information about their patients and plans for care. Students can ask questions to help clarify any concerns they may have about their responsibilities for nursing care delivery. More importantly, for faculty, preconference is a time when you can get to know your students' capabilities and their readiness to deliver nursing care. You can gain some insight into your students' thinking and possible problem areas. During preconference you may want to ask students about their patients' priority needs and their plan for organizing their time to meet these needs. Once students have shared this information with you, you can correct any student plans and offer suggestions to improve their nursing care delivery.

Postconference is a time when students and faculty can discuss the events of the clinical day. Students can analyze their clinical experiences by sharing information about their nursing care delivery and identifying problems that emerged and how they handled them. It is also a time when students can reflect on the outcomes of their nursing care and identify what they may have done differently to improve the outcomes.

The group discussions in pre- and postclinical conferences allow students to learn from their experiences. The faculty member's role is to facilitate these discussions.

Medication Administration

Medication administration is a learning activity that can enhance students' cognitive and psychomotor abilities. Students are assigned to administer medications to their patients during the clinical rotation. Faculty schedule these medication administrations and identify which students will be giving medications on any given clinical day. This information is communicated to the staff nurses as well as written on the patient assignment sheet to prevent any errors in care. When students are administering medications they need to be closely supervised by faculty or preceptors throughout the process. Because students are closely supervised during this activity, the number of students who are assigned medication administration on any given day needs to be

Box 9-1 Observational Guide

During this time, you are assigned to follow a nurse working on this unit. You will not be responsible for the delivery of nursing care, but you can assist the registered nurse if requested. While spending your time on this unit, you should be prepared to discuss the following issues/questions in clinical postconference.

Student Observational Objectives

1. Recognize the role and responsibilities of the registered nurse on this clinical unit.
2. Observe nursing care delivery systems provided to this patient population.
3. Identify systems in place to prevent patient care errors.
4. Analyze your feelings about caring for patients in this clinical setting and how these feelings may influence your care.
5. Identify discharge planning issues that may affect the patients on this unit and their families.

Student Observational Assignment

1. Compare the care administered to the patient under observation with the description of that care in the textbook.
2. Identify and explain systems used in this clinical setting to prevent patient care errors.
3. Identify at least two nursing care interventions you observed the patient receiving and explain the rationales for these interventions. How will you evaluate the effectiveness of these interventions?
4. Select one need or problem you identified for a patient you were observing and provide a rationale for it. What is an alternative need or problem you may consider, and why?
5. Identify a near miss or a potentially unsafe practice that you observed on this clinical unit. Analyze what may have gone wrong and which nursing actions were used to prevent this near miss.
6. Identify an issue that affects patient care in this setting. How would you address this issue as a charge nurse or in the role of a staff nurse?
7. Examine your feelings about caring for patients in this clinical setting. In what ways may these feelings influence your care?
8. Describe the process used in this clinical setting for medication reconciliation. How are these processes being implemented on this unit?
9. Identify discharge planning issues that may affect the patient and the family as a result of this hospitalization. Analyze these issues from two different points of view. How would you approach these issues and why? Provide a rationale for actions to be taken from both perspectives. (If there is a case manager assigned to this unit, you may want to discuss these issues with the case manager if time permits.)

limited. A faculty member may be able to supervise only one or two students administering medications on a clinical day. How many students you will assign to medication administration will also depend on the number of medications each patient needs to receive throughout the time the students are on the clinical unit. Closely supervising students during medication administration consumes much of your time as faculty and does not provide you with much time to assist the other students in the delivery of their nursing care. For this reason you need to carefully scrutinize the number of medication administrations you will assign for the clinical day. Remember, when students are assigned medication administration they need to adhere to the policies and procedures of the clinical agency.

Although opportunities to administer medications build students' skills, the process should also enhance their knowledge of medications and their ability to make decisions about when medications should be given or withheld. Faculty can promote this knowledge by having students identify the classification and action of the drug, why the patient is receiving this medication, and any nursing measures that need to be taken prior to and after the patient receives the medication.

Concept Mapping Care Plans

Concept mapping care plans are a learning activity to help nursing students plan and organize the nursing care they deliver at the clinical agency. Such a concept map is a diagram of students' ideas or "concepts" about patient problems and treatments. Students create these concept mapping care plans to organize patient data, analyze relationships in the data, and establish priorities of care. Building on students' previous knowledge, these care plans enable students to take a holistic view of their patients' situations while identifying areas where their own knowledge is limited (Schuster, 2002). Taylor and Wros (2007) write about concept mapping, "it teaches critical thinking and nursing theory, develops competence with technology, and fosters effective interchange between faculty and students" (p. 211).

However, the usefulness of concept mapping care plans as a learning strategy to enhance critical thinking and clinical reasoning among undergraduate nursing students has been found to have some methodological shortcomings (Yeo, 2014). Students themselves also have identified positive and negative experiences with the use of this learning strategy. The use of concept maps was seen as a positive experience by students who were open-minded, motivated, and visual learners. Negative experiences occurred among students who did not fully understand the purpose for concept maps and felt overwhelmed using the software needed to create the map. The time required to create the concept map and the lack of consistency among faculty when evaluating these concept maps also contributed to students' negative feelings about their use in the clinical setting (Harrison & Gibbons, 2010).

Faculty who want to use this learning strategy in the clinical setting need to consider several factors. First, faculty need to support the use of this learning strategy in the curriculum as a teaching and evaluation method. When this strategy is used throughout the curriculum, students may come to understand its purpose, thus helping to reduce learner anxiety and resistance. If concept maps are going to be used in the nursing curriculum, faculty need to attend structured workshops on the use of concept maps and their computer software applications. Once faculty are knowledgeable about the use of concept maps, they can provide the needed orientation to students and adjunct faculty. Faculty also need to be consistent when providing feedback to students to help them improve their concept maps. An evaluation tool listing the expected criteria for the concept map may need to be developed to ensure consistency in evaluation and grading.

Nursing Care Plans

Prior to the use of concept mapping, nursing care plans relied on the traditional care planning format used in undergraduate nursing schools to help students learn how to apply the nursing process when caring for patients at the clinical agency. These care plans expect students to record assessment data, identify patients' problems or needs, plan and implement interventions to address these problems or needs, and evaluate the outcomes. The linear format of this traditional method has been criticized for not encouraging the more dynamic process of critical thinking among students. With the traditional method, students may write down interventions taken from care-planning textbooks rather than thinking about individual patient data and the needs of the situation.

Despite the controversy about the use of nursing care plans to enhance critical thinking and clinical reasoning among nursing students, nursing care plans are the central facet of nursing practice (Keller, 2015). Healthcare agency accreditation groups, such as The Joint Commission, require the development of individualized care plans for every patient. These care plans provide a roadmap for patient care and include an interdisciplinary interventional approach to help achieve better patient outcomes.

Nursing students are introduced to the use of nursing care plans during their clinical practicums. The formats for these care plans differ among nursing schools, but the creation of these care plans usually follows the steps in the nursing process. These plans are intended to help students connect theory to practice. Students collect information about their patients from the patients' charts, assess their patients' needs, develop and implement a plan of care, and evaluate patient outcomes. At times, students may need to modify their plan of care to improve patient outcomes.

You may ask yourself when the best time would be for students to develop these care plans. Some nursing curricula may require faculty to assign patients to the students the day before students are to report to the clinical agency. In this situation you can have students complete the care plan before coming to the clinical site, review their care plans in preconference, and then have students present a follow-up evaluation of the care plan in postconference. When students are assigned patients on the day of the clinical experience, they are expected to develop the care plans based on the problems or needs they encountered after caring for their patients on that clinical day.

Faculty correct these care plans and return them to students with feedback identifying their strengths and weaknesses in formulating their plan of care. While correcting these care plans, faculty may also gain some insight into students' knowledge and cognitive abilities. Correcting these care plans is a time-consuming process for faculty. In some schools of nursing, a rubric for evaluating students' care plans may be available to help ensure consistency among faculty in the evaluation and grading of student assignments.

Reflective Journals

Reflective journals are another way students learn from experience through reflection. Boud (2001) examined the use of journal writing and reflection as a way to promote adult learning and concurred with Dewey's belief that reflection helps people find meaning in their personal experiences, adding that it can change conceptual perspectives and enhance personal growth.

The use of reflective journal writing as a teaching/learning strategy in undergraduate and graduate nursing curricula has become an increasing popular activity to improve students' self-awareness through reflection on learning events. When keeping a reflective journal, students express their thoughts in written form and bring this information together to create a sense of meaning about their experiences. Several outcomes have been identified as stemming from reflective journaling in nursing curricula, including professional development and empowerment among the students and faculty facilitation of the learning process (Langley & Brown, 2010).

Reflective journaling has been used as a preclass, interclass, and postclass activity to facilitate learning among nursing students (Atchison, Boatright, & Merrigan, 2006), as well as in clinical settings (Ross, 2014). In the clinical setting, the students' reflective journals need to focus on an exploration of the clinical experience and its meaning to the student. This can help faculty better understand the clinical experience from the students' perspectives and allow faculty to share perceptions, correct misconceptions, and offer insights into situations that puzzle students (O'Conner, 2006). When the purpose of the journal is to stimulate critical thinking and reflection, the assignment needs to be structured to include questions addressing students' analysis and interpretations of the situations, how they felt about the way the situation was handled, what they would have done differently to improve the outcomes, and their areas of strength and weakness that were used in this situation. If a grade is assigned to students' reflective journals, a rubric may be used that focuses on "the processes students reveal in their writings rather than the content" (O'Conner, 2006, p. 180).

Many times when students are engaged in the delivery of nursing care, their focus of learning is on the development of nursing skills needed to safely care for their patients. This only contributes to the enhancement of their motor skills. If students are required to keep a reflective journal throughout their clinical rotation, however, they are provided with opportunities to reflect on the delivery of their nursing care and patients' outcomes while considering alternative ways to improve their delivery of quality care. Subsequently, the use of reflective journaling may prompt students to use higher-order cognitive thinking and provide them with the opportunity "to think like a nurse."

Process Recordings

The process recording is a learning activity that helps students with their therapeutic communication skills and reflective learning. It can be used to evaluate students' interpersonal skills with patients in the clinical setting. Such recordings are written accounts of verbal exchanges between the patient and the student. The accounts are tied to a specific purpose, often to find out more about how patients feel about their present state of health and its effect on their lives. Students paraphrase this dialogue; analyze the interaction, identifying patients' feelings as well as their own; evaluate the effectiveness of the communication technique utilized; and summarize what was learned from using this communication technique and how they would change their patterns of communication.

Process recordings allow students to become more aware of their communication patterns with patients. By reflecting on these patterns, students may learn to improve their techniques and the quality of the communication (**Box 9-2**).

When faculty review students' process recordings they become aware of the communication techniques students tend to use in their interpersonal dialogues with patients and can offer alternative therapeutic communication techniques to improve the interaction.

Service Learning

Service learning is an active learning strategy that is becoming increasingly common in nursing education programs. It is directed at building social responsibility and civic engagement in nursing students by having these students participate in a service activity that meets community needs. This service learning project is tied to a specific nursing course and provides a way for students to connect academic learning with service, learn new skills, try new roles that encourage risk taking, and critically reflect on their service and learning experience through writings, discussions, journals, or

Box 9-2 Process Recording

Student's Name: _____ Date: _____ Duration: _____

Patient Initials: _____ Age: _____ Sex: _____

Diagnosis: _____

Description of patient's appearance at time of interaction: _____

_____

_____

Goal for the interaction: _____

Barrier to communication: _____

_____

Student's Communication	Patient's Communication	Evaluation of Communication Technique	Interpretation of Communication

class presentations (Mueller, 2009). Implementing service learning projects into the nursing curriculum was found to be a viable strategy for facilitating leadership development skills among nursing students and increasing their awareness of social justice issues present in various communities (Foli, Braswell, & Kirkpatrick, 2014; Groh, Stallwood, & Daniels, 2012).

Providing service learning experiences for students presents challenges for faculty (Ross, 2012). It is very time consuming to identify appropriate service learning situations to meet course objectives, select placement sites, plan learning activities with students and community agencies, and oversee implementation of the service learning projects. Legal issues and liability for the college and agency are also a concern whenever students perform off-campus activities related to coursework.

Legal counsel needs to be involved to ensure all contracts between the school and the agency are signed to prevent potential litigation. Several colleges and universities have service learning administrative personnel who provide assistance in structuring the project, identifying community partners, and helping with student placement in appropriate agencies. Faculty need to work closely with these service learning project administrators to ensure the learning experiences meet course objectives and learner outcomes.

THE ESSENTIALS OF BACCALAUREATE EDUCATION FOR PROFESSIONAL NURSING PRACTICE

The American Association of Colleges of Nursing (AACN, 2000) reaffirmed in 2004 its position that baccalaureate education is the minimum level required for entry into professional nursing. Several organizations, including the National League for Nursing (NLN) and the National Organization for Associate Degree Nursing, support the AACN position and advocate for associate-degree nursing graduates to continue their education toward a baccalaureate degree in nursing. In a joint statement on academic progression for associate-degree graduates into baccalaureate, master's, and doctoral programs (AACN, 2012), these educational organizations supported the need to achieve unity among nursing education programs to provide nurses with the support they need to further their nursing education.

The Essentials of Baccalaureate Education for Professional Nursing Practice (AACN, 2008) is a testimony to the importance of baccalaureate nursing education for the 21st century. This document addresses the Institute of Medicine (IOM, 2000, 2001, 2004) core competencies needed by healthcare professionals to build a safer healthcare system. *The Essentials* identifies the outcomes expected of graduates from baccalaureate nursing programs who will be practicing within complex healthcare systems as members of the profession who are providers, designers, managers, and coordinators of health care (**Table 9-3**).

A nursing faculty tool kit also developed by the AACN (2009) provides resources and exemplars to help faculty develop integrative learning strategies for classroom and clinical experiences. The tool kit provides faculty with examples of integrative learning strategies they may use when developing student assignments and projects to help meet the learner-focused outcomes. In addition to delivering hands-on nursing care in various healthcare agencies, other activities and assignments can be required in various nursing courses to satisfy learner outcomes and the essentials for baccalaureate nursing education (**Box 9-3**).

TABLE 9-3 The Essentials of Baccalaureate Education for Professional Nursing Practice (2008)

Baccalaureate Essentials	Practice-Focused Outcomes
I. Liberal Education for Baccalaureate Generalist Nursing Practice	A solid base in liberal education provides the cornerstone for the practice and education of nurses.
II. Basic Organizational and Systems Leadership for Quality Care and Patient Safety	Knowledge and skills in leadership, quality improvement, and patient safety are necessary to provide high-quality care.
III. Scholarship for Evidence-Based Practice	Professional nursing practice is grounded in the translation of current evidence into practice.
IV. Information Management and Application of Patient Care Technology	Knowledge and skills in information management and patient care technology are critical in the delivery of quality patient care.
V. Healthcare Policy, Finance, and Regulatory Environments	Healthcare policies, including financial and regulatory, directly and indirectly influence the nature and functioning of the healthcare system and therefore are important considerations in professional nursing practice.
VI. Interprofessional Communication and Collaboration for Improving Patient Health Outcomes	Communication and collaboration among healthcare professionals are critical to delivering high-quality and safe patient care.
VII. Clinical Prevention and Population Health for Optimizing Health	Health promotion and disease prevention at the individual and population levels are necessary to improve population health and are important components of baccalaureate generalist nursing practice.
VIII. Professionalism and Professional Values	Professionalism and the inherent values of altruism, autonomy, human dignity, integrity, and social justice are fundamental to nursing.
IX. Baccalaureate Generalist Nursing Practice	The baccalaureate-graduate nurse is prepared to practice with patients, including individuals, families, groups, communities, and populations across the lifespan and across the continuum of healthcare communities. The baccalaureate graduate understands and respects the variations of care, the increased complexity, and the increased use of healthcare resources inherent in caring for patients.

Reproduced from American Association of Colleges of Nursing. (2008). *The essentials of baccalaureate education for professional nursing practice*. Washington, DC: Author. Retrieved from http://www.aacn.nche.edu/education-resources/Bacc Essentials08.pdf

---

Box 9-3 Learner Assignments/Activities

- Develop safety and quality improvement projects for diverse populations.
- Create evidence-based research papers about healthcare delivery topics.
- Attend political forums addressing healthcare policy and finance.
- Write position papers on various healthcare topics.
- Participate in collaborative projects to enhance quality improvement.
- Participate in interdisciplinary forums to improve communication among all healthcare providers.
- Shadow a leader in a healthcare agency to identify leadership skills, organizational processes, and system-related patient care problems.
- Use simulation labs to engage in interprofessional and intraprofessional healthcare delivery.
- Use case-based scenarios to apply the nursing process among culturally diverse patient populations.
- Engage in service learning activities to promote wellness in the community across the lifespan.
- Participate in and report about quality improvement activities focused on patient care delivery methods, regulatory requirements, and information systems.
- Perform community- or population-focused assessments and develop plans to address the health issues identified in the community.
- Write intensive assignments to promote reflection on individuals' own beliefs and values about various moral/ethical issues such as right-to-die, do not resuscitate (DNR) orders, and patient advocacy.

Essential I, Liberal Education for Baccalaureate Generalist Practice, recognizes the need for nurses to have a solid base in liberal education. Studying the humanities, social sciences, and natural sciences provides a broad exposure to multiple disciplines and ways of knowing. Completion of courses in liberal education forms the basis for intellectual inquiry, analysis, critical thinking, communication, and cultural awareness. A liberal education also enhances the development of personal value systems, ethical decision making, leadership skills, and a responsibility to promote social justice. Liberal education prepares nurses to face the challenges of today's changing healthcare system by forming the foundation of their professional values and standards.

To operationalize this essential into the nursing curriculum, the tool kit provides several learning activities faculty may use to meet practice-focused outcomes. Faculty may choose opportunities or assignments for students that:

- Provide local, national, and international experiences, framed by reflective questions, in a variety of cultures, organizations, and communities

- Promote activities and projects with students from the arts, humanities, and sciences to address community issues or problems
- Use collaborative learning projects to build communication and leadership skills
- Engage in community-based activities to promote ethical reasoning, advocacy, collaboration, and social justice
- Provide opportunities to reflect on one's own actions and values to promote ongoing self-assessment and commitment to excellence in practice
- Provide guided exploration of diverse philosophies, ways of knowing, and intellectual approaches to problem solving
- Use simulation exercises and case-based scenarios with students from other academic disciplines such as history, religion, business, and engineering
- Provide direct experiences integrating artistic ways of knowing such as the arts, cinema, poetry, literature, and music to enhance the practice of nursing
- Provide opportunities to observe and participate in various cultures through study abroad
- Participate in interprofessional service learning activities such as health promotion and disease prevention projects for diverse populations
- Use writing-intensive assignments to promote reflection, insight, and integration of ideas across disciplines and courses (AACN, 2009)

Essential II, Basic Organizational and Systems Leadership for Quality Care and Patient Safety, recognizes the need for professional nurses to have knowledge of organizational and systems leadership, quality improvement measures, and safety principles to deliver high-quality patient care. To operationalize this essential into the nursing curriculum, the tool kit provides several learning activities faculty may use to meet practice-focused outcomes. Faculty may choose assignments that provide opportunities for students to:

- Engage in leadership experiences in a variety of organizations and communities to build communication and leadership skills
- Communicate with recognized leaders to solve healthcare practice problems
- Develop a leadership or quality improvement project that spans several courses
- Shadow a leader and reflect on the experience
- Engage in quality improvement/patient safety activities to promote an understanding of the organizational process, unit application, and evaluation process
- Participate in quality improvement activities and/or required regulatory reporting systems
- Participate in an interprofessional performance improvement team currently working on implementation/evaluation of national patient safety goals
- Propose an innovative solution to a system-related patient care problem identified in one's clinical practice

- Conduct a mock root-cause analysis on a near miss and share results with staff or shared governance council
- Participate in an actual root-cause analysis (RCA) and/or failure mode effects analysis (FMEA)
- Role-play with nursing and medical students using situation, background, assessment, recommendation (SBAR) communication
- Attend a professional nursing organization meeting and identify personal development opportunities
- Examine various microsystem committees, and identify one for more in-depth exploration (AACN, 2009)

Essential III, Scholarship for Evidence-Based Practice, supports the need for scientific evidence when identifying practice issues, and the interpretation and integration of reliable evidence to inform practice and improve patient outcomes. To operationalize this essential into the curriculum, assignments may include the following:

- Ask students to select a clinical topic, search for evidence, and identify the level of evidence for each sample of evidence.
- Create journal clubs where students critique a primary nursing research article and its relevance to their clinical practice.
- Group students according to a clinical issue of interest, conduct a systematic review, and debate the rigor of selected research studies.
- Use controversial case studies to promote discussion about decision making and the evidence that supports those decisions.
- Collaborate with librarians to conduct comprehensive and efficient searches on clinical topics.
- Provide a sample of nursing journals and ask students to identify a research article and determine the type and level of evidence included.
- Assign student peer review of a student colleague's paper.
- Identify clinical questions in PICO (patient problem, intervention, compare, outcome) format and conduct searches for current evidence using the PubMed PICO search feature.
- Examine the evidence for an existing policy or procedure using multiple sources (e.g., Cochrane, AHRQ, CINAHL, PubMed).
- Apply specific criteria to evaluate health information resources for lay and professional use as well as to discuss the ethical implications of commercial sources that target laypersons.
- Collaborate with clinical partners to identify practice problems, formulate evidence-based conclusions and recommendations, and present findings in poster format to staff and class.
- Apply evidence-based practice models to assess the applicability and feasibility of new findings to practice.

- Cite sources of evidence for planned interventions.
- For assigned patients, compare observed practices with published practice standards.
- Link how individual nursing actions are related to recognized nurse sensitive quality indicators. (AACN, 2009)

Essential IV, Information Management and Application of Patient Care Technology, recognizes the need for nurses to have a basic level of competency in nursing informatics and be able to use patient care computer applications and information management systems in the delivery of patient care. Nurses will use these information management systems to document patient care and communicate across multiple healthcare disciplines. Assignments included in the tool kit to operationalize this essential include the following:

- Use information and patient care technology to communicate effectively with members of the healthcare team.
- Use clinical evidence and research to base and validate practice decisions related to information management and patient care technology.
- Participate in quality improvement activities and required regulatory reporting through information systems.
- Employ a range of technologies that support patient care, such as electronic health and medical records, patient monitoring systems, and medication administration systems.
- Use simulation and electronic medical records to access and analyze data relevant to the patient situation.
- Use information technology resources such as Wiki, Second Life simulation, or SkyScape.com to communicate with other healthcare professionals or students in other disciplines regarding a joint project.
- Develop a professional e-portfolio. (AACN, 2009)

Essential V, Healthcare Policy, Finance, and Regulatory Environments, supports the need for nurses to have a broad understanding of healthcare policies, including financial and regulatory policies, that directly affect patient care. This includes knowledge of how patient care services are organized, financed, and reimbursed. Nurses also need to participate in political areas as advocates for their patients, families, and vulnerable communities, and as voices for change regarding nursing's role in changing the healthcare delivery system. Tool kit exemplars that help operationalize this essential into the curriculum include the following:

- Observe a state board of nursing hearing and reflect on how the state practice act protects the welfare and safety of the state's citizens.
- Participate with national or state nursing associations in activities such as "lobby day."

- Review proposed legislation affecting health care and provide written comments.
- Attend national or state congressional hearings on healthcare issues.
- Observe testimony at a state legislative or regulatory hearing on a healthcare issue focusing on access to care or patient advocacy.
- Provide written or verbal feedback on the ethical, financial, and social implications of the testimony observed and recommended policy changes.
- Compare the costs of common diagnostic tests, procedures, and medications charged to insurance companies versus self-pay patients.
- Explore the costs and availability of care options for patients with dementia or a psychiatric/mental health illness in your local community. (What does private health insurance cover? Medicaid? Medicare?)
- Develop a lobbying plan for an identified issue that includes a concise (30 seconds or less) oral synopsis for a decision maker and a one-page policy memo.
- Participate in advocating for a change in policy related to a selected healthcare issue at the local, state, or national level.
- As an interprofessional group, role play a legislator, proponent, and opponent for a healthcare or professional issue.
- Analyze a hospital bill for one day of care in an acute setting and identify where nursing services are embedded.
- Compare one or more healthcare systems in other countries with the U.S. system, including costs, services provided, and outcomes (e.g., prenatal and postnatal care, role of midwife and other healthcare professionals/workers, insurance coverage, maternity/paternity leave).
- As an interprofessional group, develop a policy (new or revised) to address an issue identified in a practice setting. Delineate processes for getting the policy adopted and implemented within that practice setting. (AACN, 2009)

Essential VI, Interprofessional Communication and Collaboration for Improving Patient Health Outcomes, advocates for the need to have effective communication and collaboration among all healthcare professionals to deliver quality patient-centered care. This requires effective teamwork, with interprofessional and intraprofessional collaboration around shared goals, role expectations, decision-making processes, communication, and leadership. This essentially helps to establish respect and trust among all members of the healthcare team. Tool kit assignments or opportunities to help operationalize this essential into the curriculum include the following:

- Engage in case study discussions/dialogue with a variety of healthcare and other professionals.
- Participate in interprofessional collaboration (e.g., grand rounds, community coalition meetings).

- Work in interprofessional and intraprofessional teams on course projects/assignments.
- Engage in interprofessional and intraprofessional care in simulation labs.
- Develop interprofessional community projects.
- Assess the group dynamics of an interprofessional or intraprofessional group. After attending a professional meeting of another healthcare profession, compare and contrast professional perspectives.
- Participate in interprofessional teams at national competitions.
- Participate in campus-wide student governance and committees.
- Organize activities for National Primary Care Week as a student ambassador. (AACN, 2009)

Essential VII, Clinical Prevention and Population Health for Optimizing Health, identifies health promotion and disease and injury prevention as needed components in the nursing curriculum. The delivery of health promotion and disease prevention efforts by nurses is important throughout the lifespan of individuals, families, groups, and communities and during times of disasters. In this population-focused nursing, nurses require knowledge about growth and development, evidence-based prevention strategies, immunization practices, health teaching, and counseling. Nurses need to be attentive to the effectiveness, efficiency, cost-effectiveness, and equity of population-focused interventions while advocating for healthcare policies that promote health and prevent disease. To meet this essential, opportunities or assignments for students should include the following:

- Analyze health behavior(s) of self or others using models or theories.
- Participate in individually focused clinical prevention activities such as:
  - Teaching about and providing immunizations
  - Improving adherence to tuberculosis chemoprophylaxis through health teaching and directly observed therapies
  - Providing health counseling regarding smoking cessation, stress management, exercise, and diet
  - Teaching about and encouraging cancer screening
  - Conducting basic environmental exposure history regarding pesticides
  - Conducting basic genetic health screening and referring high-risk individuals to genetic services
  - Assessing a home environment and health counseling to prevent falls in older adults
  - Identifying and intervening in elder abuse
- Use clinical practice guidelines for planning and/or evaluating clinical prevention interventions.

- Participate in community- or population-focused assessment.
- Participate in the development of plans and policies to effectively prepare a community for disasters or to protect vulnerable populations during disasters.
- Help organizations and communities create healthy environments such as smoke-free workplaces.
- Teach vulnerable populations about avoiding environmental risks.
- Collaborate with institutions, such as daycare centers or homeless shelters, to develop and implement policies to minimize transmission of communicable diseases.
- Participate in a community disaster drill.
- Develop a policy memo to address a health issue identified in the community.
- Advocate for policy change regarding a health issue identified in the community.
- Initiate an interprofessional going-green campaign to improve environmental health. (AACN, 2009)

Essential VIII, Professionalism and Professional Values, includes an understanding of the historical, legal, and contemporary contexts of nursing practice. Nurses are expected to apply the principles of altruism, excellence, caring, ethics, respect, communication, and accountability in the delivery of nursing care. As professionals, nurses are accountable for their own actions and maintain a continuous professional involvement in lifelong learning. Nurses have professional values that guide their ability to make decisions within the context of their patients' values. Ethics and honesty are an integral part of professional practice when advocating for the rights and needs of patients. To operationalize these beliefs and values, assignments and opportunities may include the following:

- Write a letter to the editor or opinion editorial about the role of nursing in improving health care, and submit the letter to a local newspaper for publication.
- Observe and respond to focused questions about the proceedings of ethical review committees, institutional review boards (IRBs), nursing practice councils, and state boards of nursing meetings and/or hearings.
- Participate in professional- or community-based organizations that advocate for quality and access to care.
- Use simulated vignettes that address ethical, legal, and moral patient care situations such as:
  - Provider abandonment of a patient
  - Decision making about reporting to work in the event of a disaster
  - Reporting sexual assault or abuse
  - Suspected drug use by a colleague
  - End-of-life decision making

- Identification of a spiritual crisis
- Withdrawal of life support

- Participate in interprofessional service learning projects such as student visits to secondary schools, school career days, summer health camps, or vulnerable populations in homeless shelters or homes for battered women and children.
- Partner with a nursing school from another country to gain a global perspective; use the Internet to obtain global experiences.
- Engage in legislative state house visits to articulate the professional nursing role/ perspective.
- Work with legislative staff at various levels.
- Participate in rounds with chaplains or other spiritual care professionals.
- Develop a self-care improvement plan. For example, use a tool such as the "Circle of Human Potentials" (Dossey & Keegan, 2009) to conduct a self-assessment and develop a self-care improvement plan that includes measurable outcomes.
- Conduct a self-assessment in one or more of the following areas: physical, emotional, spiritual, cultural, relationships, communications, and learning style. Based on this assessment, develop an improvement plan that includes measurable outcomes.
- Analyze the media's portrayal of nurses and other aspects of health care.
- Discuss cultural and ethical variables in patient care scenarios using software, such as The Neighborhood (Gidden, 2007), in interprofessional/intraprofessional learning groups.
- Use reflective writing to discuss student use of moral agency and/or patient advocacy.
- Create a student honor code to be adopted.
- Engage with a nurse actively involved in professional nursing practice for more than 30 years to explore changes within the profession. (AACN, 2009)

Essential IX, Baccalaureate Generalist Nursing Practice, integrates the knowledge, skills, and abilities critical to professional nursing practice and delineated in Essentials I–VIII. Nurses practice in various healthcare settings and across the lifespan using the nursing process to guide patient care and promote a therapeutic nurse–patient relationship. To operationalize this essential into the nursing curriculum, the tool kit provides several learning activities that faculty may use to meet practice-focused outcomes. They include the following:

- In a group of students, plan, provide, and evaluate nursing care for a patient with multiple comorbidities and symptoms in a simulated or patient care environment.
- In a group of interprofessional students, provide care that reflects patient preferences and values in a simulated or patient care environment.

- Arrange cultural immersion caregiving experiences in settings such as homeless shelters, migrant clinics, correctional facilities, and corporate health settings.
- Provide evidence-based, patient-centered end-of-life care to a dying patient and his or her significant others.
- Interview volunteers with complex problems, such as human immunodeficiency virus (HIV), psychiatric conditions, tuberculosis, or substance abuse to explore patient preferences and values.
- Provide care to a group of patients that incorporates delegation, supervision, and outcomes evaluation.
- Administer and document administration of medications to groups of patients in a patient care or simulated environment.
- Perform patient assessment and evaluation of a patient's response to pharmacological agents in a simulated or patient care environment.
- Use unfolding case study analysis to correlate a patient's medical condition and pathophysiology, and design appropriate therapeutic interventions.
- Use a constructed genetic pedigree from collected family history information to identify a risk profile and develop a plan of care, including patient education and referral.
- Use simulation, case studies, and patient assignments to make decisions about the organization, prioritization, and appropriate delegation of care.
- Consult with other professionals to improve transitions of elderly patients across care settings.
- Evaluate patient education materials for cultural and linguistic appropriateness.
- Elicit a spiritual history and integrate a patient's spirituality into the care plan.[1]

Although these *Essentials* are for baccalaureate nursing education, they apply to all prelicensure and RN completion programs. Faculty from associate-degree nursing programs need to include these *Essentials* into their curriculum development efforts if they want to help with the progression of nursing students' achievement of the learner-focused outcomes of the baccalaureate nursing degree. If you are a faculty member developing courses in an associate-degree program, you may not have time to include all nine essentials in the program. Faculty do not need to develop a separate course for each essential. Instead, specific courses can be designed to address more than one essential to achieve the practice-focused outcome. For example, when an assignment is developed to address Essential I, Liberal Education, the cultural needs of patient populations can be addressed in medical–surgical, obstetrics, pediatrics, community, and leadership courses. Remember, all learning opportunities that faculty provide for students, including direct clinical experiences, should focus on developing and applying

---

[1]Courtesy of AACN.

the knowledge, skills, and abilities necessary to manage care and achieve the learner-focused outcomes defined in the *Essentials*.

SUMMARY

This chapter explored the application of experiential learning theory in the clinical setting to achieve the IOM and QSEN competencies required for the delivery of quality health care. Various clinical learning strategies used by faculty to develop the knowledge, skills, and abilities required by beginning practitioners were presented. Organizing student learning experiences in clinical agencies and strategies to promote critical thinking and clinical reasoning were also discussed. Finally, *The Essentials for Baccalaureate Education for Professional Nursing Practice* were presented together with a tool kit of assignments or activities that faculty may implement to operationalize these *Essentials* in the clinical setting.

CASE STUDIES

1. This is your first job as a clinical educator, and you are taking a clinical group of 10 sophomore nursing students to a medical–surgical unit in an acute care hospital for a 15-week clinical rotation.
   - Design the agenda for your first clinical preconference.
   - Design the agenda for your first clinical postconference.
   - Discuss how you would decide the learning activities for these students, and create the patient care assignment for each of these students.
2. You have assigned a fourth-level student to a 72-year-old male patient admitted to the acute care hospital with abdominal pain, fever, and altered mental status. The patient's history includes alcohol abuse, pancreatitis, cardiomyopathy, and renal failure. Create a written assignment to evaluate the student's application of the nursing process.
3. You have assigned an observational experience to one of the students in your clinical group. This student will spend the day in the surgical intensive care unit. Identify the student observational objectives for this experience, and develop a list of criteria for this student to share in postconference.
4. You are a clinical faculty member assigned to a homeless shelter for three weeks. Four students are assigned to come to this agency each week. Referring to *The Essentials of Baccalaureate Education for Nursing Practice*:
   - Design learning activities for these students.
   - Choose one or two *Essentials* and create written assignments for these students in this healthcare agency that operationalize achievement of the *Essentials*.

REFERENCES

American Association of Colleges of Nursing (AACN). (2000). *The baccalaureate degree in nursing as minimal preparation for professional practice.* Washington, DC: Author. Retrieved from http://www.aacn.nche.edu/publications/position/bacc-degree-prep

American Association of Colleges of Nursing (AACN). (2008). *The essentials of baccalaureate education for professional nursing practice.* Washington, DC: Author. Retrieved from http://www.aacn.nche.edu/education-resources/BaccEssentials08.pdf

American Association of Colleges of Nursing (AACN). (2009). *Nursing faculty tool kit for the implementation of the baccalaureate essentials.* Washington, DC: Author. Retrieved from http://www.aacn.nche.edu/education-resources/BacEssToolkit.pdf

American Association of Colleges of Nursing (AACN). (2012). *Joint statement on academic progression for nursing students and graduates.* Washington, DC: Author. Retrieved from http://www.aacn.nche.edu/aacn-publications/position/joint-statement-academic-progression

Atchison, C., Boatright, D., & Merrigan, D. Demonstrating excellence in practice-based teaching for public health. *Journal of Public Health Practice and Management, 12*(1), 15–21.

Boud, D. (2001). Using journal writing to enhance reflective practice. *New Direction for Adult and Continuing Education, 90,* 9–17.

Cell, E. (1984). *Learning to learn from experience.* Albany, NY: State University of New York.

Cronenwett, L., Sherwood, G., Barnsteiner, J., Disch, J., Johnson, J., Mitchell, P., Sullivan, D. T., & Warren, J. (2007). Quality and safety education for nurses. *Nursing Outlook, 55,* 122–131.

Daley, B. J. (2001). Learning in clinical practice. *Holistic Nursing Practice, 16*(1), 43–54.

Dewey, J. (1933). *How we think.* Boston, MA: D. C. Heath.

Dewey, J. (1938). *Experience and education.* New York, NY: Collier.

Dossey, B. M., & Keegan, L. (2009). *Holistic nursing: A handbook for practice* (6th ed.). Sudbury, MA: Jones and Bartlett Publishers.

Foli, K. J., Braswell, M., & Kirkpatrick, J. (2014). Development of leadership behaviors in undergraduate nursing students: A service learning approach. *Nursing Education Perspectives, 35*(2), 76–82.

Gaberson, K. B., & Oermann, M. H. (2010). *Clinical teaching strategies in nursing* (3rd ed.). New York, NY: Springer.

Giddens, J. F. (2007). The neighborhood. *Nursing Education Perspective, 28*(5), 251–256.

Gron, C. J., Stallwood, L. G., & Daniels, J. J. (2011). Service-learning in nursing education: Its impact on leadership and social justice. *Nursing Education Perspectives, 32*(6), 400–405.

Harrison, S., & Gibbons, C. (2010). Nursing student perceptions of concept maps: From theory to practice. *Nursing Education Perspectives, 34*(6), 395–399.

Institute of Medicine (IOM). (2000). *To err is human: Building a safer health system.* Washington, DC: National Academies Press.

Institute of Medicine (IOM). (2001). *Crossing the quality chasm.* Washington, DC: National Academies Press.

Institute of Medicine (IOM). (2004). *Keeping patients safe: Transforming the work environment of nurses.* Washington, DC: National Academies Press.

Jarvis, P. (1987). *Adult learning in a social context.* London, UK: Croom Helm.

Keller, M. (2015, Summer). Nursing care plans are an essential part of scope of practice. *Minnesota Nursing Accent, 12.*

Langley, M., & Brown, S. T. (2010). Perceptions of the use of reflective learning journals in online graduate nursing education. *Nursing Education Perspectives, 31*(1), 12–17.

Mueller, C. (2009). Service learning: Developing values and social responsibilities. In D. M. Billings & J. A. Halstead (Eds.), *Teaching in nursing: A guide for faculty* (3rd ed., pp. 173–185). St. Louis, MO: Elsevier/Saunders.

O'Connor, A. (2006). *Clinical instruction and evaluation.* Sudbury, MA: Jones and Bartlett Publishers.

Ross, C. (2014). Evaluation of nursing students' work experience through the use of reflective journals. *Mental Health Practice, 17*(60), 21–27.

Ross, M. E. T. (2012). Linking classroom learning to the community through service learning. *Journal of Community Health Nursing, 29*(1), 53–60.

Schon, D. A. (1983). *The reflective practitioner*. New York, NY: Basic.

Schuster. P. M. (2002). *Concept mapping: A critical approach to care planning*. Philadelphia, PA: FA Davis.

Stokes, L., & Kost, G. (2009). Teaching in the clinical setting. In D. M. Billings & J. A. Halstead (Eds.), *Teaching in nursing: A guide for faculty* (3rd ed., pp. 291–292). St. Louis, MO: Saunders.

Taylor, J., & Wros, P. (2007). Concept mapping: A nursing model for care planning. *Journal of Nursing Education, 46*(5), 211–215.

Wachter, R. (2010). Patient safety at ten: Unmistakable progress, troubling gaps. *Health Affairs, 29*(1), 1–8.

Yeo, C. M. (2014). Concept mapping: A strategy to improve critical thinking. *Singapore Journal of Nursing, 41*(3), 2–8.

CHAPTER 10

Evaluating the Clinical Experience

OBJECTIVES

- Examine the clinical evaluation process and how it is used to evaluate students' performance in the clinical setting.
- Identify the challenges faced by faculty involved in the evaluation of clinical practice.
- Examine the importance of providing effective feedback to students in the clinical setting.
- Employ constructive feedback techniques.
- Utilize various data collection methods to evaluate students' overall performance in the clinical setting.
- Explain faculty responsibilities with students who are at risk for failing the clinical course.
- Create a clinical evaluation tool with expected student behaviors and grading scales that measure clinical objectives or core competencies.

The evaluation of nursing students' clinical performance is a challenging responsibility for nursing faculty. Unlike classroom evaluation, which is grounded in objective testing strategies to measure cognitive achievements, clinical evaluation is more subjective in nature and requires faculty to evaluate students' affective and psychomotor skills in addition to judging their ability to deliver safe, knowledgeable nursing care to patients. Clinical evaluation is designed to determine whether students achieve the core competencies and program outcomes required by nurses to practice safely as beginning practitioners. Therefore, evaluation of students' clinical performance needs to be reliable, valid, and accurate because these evaluations will determine whether students succeed in the nursing program.

This chapter will explore the multidimensional aspects of clinical evaluation, challenges faced by nursing faculty responsible for clinical evaluation, and strategies that address ways to strengthen evaluation methods to ensure your graduates are equipped with the knowledge, skills, and abilities necessary to work safely as beginning practitioners.

CLINICAL EVALUATION: WHAT IS IT ALL ABOUT?

Clinical evaluation in nursing education is an important responsibility of nursing faculty that has serious implications for students, faculty, and the recipients of nursing care. The word *evaluation* refers to a process of systematically and objectively judging the value, worth, and merit of someone or something in a careful and thoughtful way (Scriven, 1991). In the clinical setting, faculty are expected to judge whether students can safely and effectively implement patient care in real-life situations. The clinical setting is also where faculty provide opportunities for students to develop the standards of competence and expertise needed by beginning practitioners. Therefore, clinical evaluation seeks to determine whether students have acquired the cognitive, affective, and psychomotor skills required to meet the clinical outcome objectives defined by the school of nursing.

However, there is a lack of consistency among schools of nursing in the expected clinical outcome objectives and how they are measured. This lack of consistency in expected outcomes is due to variations in clinical settings where students are given their learning experiences, differences in patient populations and their nursing care needs, and disparity among faculty's personal perceptions and instincts about student expectations in the clinical setting. This need to evaluate the safety and competency of nursing students in the clinical setting requires closing the gap among these variations and inconsistencies. There need to be standardized clinical outcomes, and valid and reliable instruments with which to measure these outcomes (Holaday & Buckley, 2008).

Clinical evaluation is not the same as grading classroom exams. Evaluation of students' performance involves subjective and objective appraisal. Clinical evaluation is mostly subjective because it requires faculty observation of student behaviors and clinical performance to judge students' ability to deliver safe care. Clinical evaluations also are amenable to objective evaluation when evaluating students' ability to correctly follow the steps in a procedure—for example, medication administration. Because clinical evaluation is mostly a process where judgments are made by faculty about students' competencies in the clinical environment, these judgments may be biased by the faculty's value systems and influence the inferences and conclusions you make about students' performances in the clinical setting. For this reason, it is important for faculty to be aware of their own values that may bias their judgment of students. For example, if a faculty member values students who are self-starters in the clinical setting, this value should not influence the evaluation of the student's competencies in other areas (Gaberson & Oermann, 2015).

The ultimate goal of clinical evaluation is to determine whether a student is demonstrating an acceptable level of clinical performance throughout the nursing program. For this reason, clinical evaluation should be based on clinical objectives or competencies. Without this, faculty do not have any criteria for evaluating student performance, and students do not have any basis for knowing their strengths and limitations. For example, the Quality and Safety Education for Nurses (QSEN) competencies of Patient-Centered Care, Teamwork and Collaboration, Evidence-Based Practice, Quality Improvement, Safety, Informatics, and Professionalism can be used as a framework for evaluating students' abilities in the clinical setting. Expanding on the QSEN competency model is the Massachusetts Nurse of the Future Core Competency Model (Sroczynski, Gravil, Route, Hoffart, & Creelmann, 2010). Both the QSEN and Nurse of the Future (NOF) competency models are congruent with the Institute of Medicine (IOM) core competencies for all areas of health care. When students' clinical performance is compared to these core competencies, there exists a criterion-referenced interpretation of the evaluation process that may contribute to the validity and reliability of the evaluation instrument. When these core competencies are used to evaluate student behaviors in the clinical setting, students know what is expected from them and how they will meet these competencies.

Separate evaluation tools are needed for each clinical rotation. Each of these evaluation tools identifies the clinical objectives or core competencies specific for the nursing course and the behaviors expected from students to satisfy the course objectives or clinical competencies.

Clinical evaluations can be formative or summative. Formative evaluation by faculty in the clinical setting provides feedback to students regarding the progress they are making toward meeting the clinical objectives and core competencies. This form of evaluation continues throughout the clinical rotation to help students develop further in their clinical knowledge, skills, and abilities. This is also a time for faculty to provide constructive feedback to help students improve their performance. Clinical faculty need to provide these constructive suggestions to students when they observe student behaviors that do not align with the core competencies. For example, suppose you observe a student administering medications through a feeding tube, and the student has not determined placement of the tube prior to giving the medication. At this point the medication administration should be stopped and you should provide feedback or ask the student about the safety precautions needed prior to administering medications through a feeding tube. Because formative evaluation is diagnostic of students' abilities, it is not graded. Instead, this form of assessment is done to improve students' performance in the future when they need to administer medication through a feeding tube. Thus, the overall goal of formative evaluation is to improve students' performance throughout their clinical practicum.

Summative clinical evaluation is not diagnostic, but instead summarizes the student's clinical performance at the end of the clinical rotation. The goal of summative evaluation is to judge the extent to which the student has met the clinical objectives or core competencies. Summative evaluation comes at the end of a clinical rotation, so it is too late for students to improve their performance. For this reason, clinical faculty continually need to do formative evaluation throughout the clinical rotation to help students improve their clinical performance and receive a passing grade on their summative evaluation. How much formative evaluation should faculty do throughout the clinical rotation before making the final judgment about a student's ability to safely deliver nursing care without continuous help from the faculty? At what point do faculty judge a student's behaviors as satisfying or not satisfying core competencies and clinical objectives? These are challenging questions for faculty to address. Grading is the final outcome of summative evaluation and the clinical evaluation process. The grade given to students may be either a pass/fail or A through F grade. However, faculty need sufficient data about students' clinical performance before judging whether students' behaviors have met core competencies and assigning a grade. This topic will be presented in more depth later in this chapter.

CHALLENGES FOR NURSING FACULTY

Clinical evaluation of nursing students is a daunting, complex, and problematic task for faculty because it requires the direct observation of students engaged in actual practice in unpredictable clinical environments (Benner, 1982). These observations are highly subjective because of observer bias, resulting in a lack of consistency among the scores given by evaluators and the quality of the data collected. To achieve standards of competence in the clinical setting, Oermann and Gaberson (2014) believe there is a need for a valid and reliable mechanism to determine whether students can apply the knowledge learned in the classroom to implementing safe and effective patient care in real-life situations. Several research studies have been undertaken to develop an efficient and reliable evaluation tool that measures the clinical performance of undergraduate nursing students and assesses the critical competencies students must demonstrate in the clinical setting (Karayurt, Mert, & Beser, 2008; Parra et al., 2015).

Clinical evaluation is also complicated by the fact that faculty have many seemingly incompatible roles in the clinical environment, such as mentor, participant-observer, and judge or gatekeeper, when assuming the responsibility for deciding whether students' clinical performances satisfy clinical objectives and core competencies. These dual roles of faculty as educators and evaluators have been reconciled by viewing the evaluation process as having dual purposes—namely, to educate students and to judge their clinical abilities. In the clinical setting, the evaluation process is educative because faculty are responsible for overseeing the nursing care delivered by students and providing needed information to improve the teaching/learning process. This is referred to as the formative purpose of evaluation. In addition, the evaluation process has a judging or gatekeeping function because faculty are responsible for making definitive judgments about students' abilities to maintain professional practice standards and for protecting the public by ensuring students are qualified to practice as novice nurses prepared to deliver safe, quality care (Mahara, 1998). This can be referred to as the summative purpose of clinical evaluation.

Another challenge for faculty involved in clinical evaluation is the complexity of the evaluation process itself. Evaluation requires a systematic collection and interpretation of data gathered from multiple sources about students' clinical competencies. Once these data are collected, faculty make the decision as to whether students have passed the course. This faculty decision involves objective and subjective judgments about students' abilities to meet acceptable standards of practice; however, as previously stated, there is no one agreed-upon definition or consistent standard for evaluation of clinical competence (Edmond, 2001; Skingley, Arnott, Graves, & Nabb, 2006).

To address the many problems of consistency and reliability in the evaluation of student outcomes in the clinical setting, several standardized assessment and evaluation instruments have been developed that seek evidence-based knowledge of students in real-life situations and are based on clinical outcomes recognized by the profession. These evaluation tool kits were developed to improve the accuracy and reliability of the clinical evaluation process by reducing discrepancies among evaluators while assessing the growth in students' performances throughout the nursing program (Holaday & Buckley, 2004; Reising & Devich, 2004; Walsh et al., 2010).

Although the clinical evaluation process presents challenges for faculty, the evaluation process needs to be fair. To establish a fair evaluation process, Gaberson and Oermann (2010) provide the following suggestions:

- Faculty need to identify their own values, attitudes, beliefs, and biases and realize how these may influence their evaluation of students.
- Clinical evaluation needs to be based on predetermined core competencies or clinical objectives.
- Faculty need to develop a supportive clinical learning environment where students feel comfortable seeking assistance from faculty who provide constructive feedback.

Although the evaluation process presents challenges for faculty, faculty need to work together to develop an evaluation process that is fair, consistent, and related to course objectives and clinical competencies.

PROVIDING FEEDBACK IN CLINICAL EVALUATION

Research by John Hattie (2008) revealed that feedback was among the most powerful influences on achievement. The term *feedback* is often used to describe the advice, praise, or evaluation given to individuals about how they are doing in their efforts to reach a goal. Providing feedback to students in the clinical setting to help them improve performance is an important responsibility of faculty. Without this help from faculty, students will have a difficult time achieving the clinical objectives. Students need to feel that faculty are there to facilitate their learning and achievement of the clinical competencies. For this reason, faculty need to develop a supportive learning environment that encourages students to ask questions and seek their help. Students need to feel comfortable identifying their limitations, knowing faculty are there to help them move forward rather than criticize them for these limitations. Years of education research have concluded that if faculty teach less and provide more feedback, students achieve greater learning (Bransford, Brown, & Cocking, 2000; Dean, Hubbell, Pitler, & Stone, 2012).

Feedback is useful for identifying when students' performances are going in the right direction or for indicating when their performances need to be redirected. The reason faculty give feedback is to provide students with the useful guidance needed to support effective behaviors that contribute to core competencies or to help them get back on track performing the correct behaviors that will meet clinical objectives. This action by faculty is known as constructive feedback. For example, you may need to provide specific performance pointers to help students correctly demonstrate a skill needed for the safe delivery of patient care, or you may need to provide corrective guidance after a skill is performed. You also need to have ongoing performance discussions with your students to let them know if they are moving in the right direction toward meeting clinical objectives, as well as to let them know the consequences if their future performances continue to not meet clinical objectives or core competencies. You should observe for certain clues in students' performances to help you know when feedback is necessary. For example, if unresolved problems persist, students continue to make the same errors repeatedly, and the nursing care they administer to their patients does not meet expectations, feedback is needed from the instructor.

Part of being an effective clinical instructor is knowing when and how to give feedback that is constructive and useful to build student confidence and trusting relationships. Learning to give constructive feedback will take time and effort on your part as a clinical faculty member. Wiggins (2012) identified the following seven keys to effective feedback (see **Box 10-1**).

Constructive feedback needs to be goal-referenced. When providing constructive feedback, you need to focus on the description of the behavior that has occurred and not judge this behavior as "right or wrong" or "good or bad." You need to avoid this evaluative language because students are likely to respond defensively. For example, "When administrating medications you checked four of the five rights; however, you did not identify the patient before giving him the medications. Patients need to be identified before medications are administered."

> **Box 10-1** Seven Keys to Effective Feedback
>
> - Goal-referenced
> - Tangible and transparent
> - Actionable
> - User-friendly
> - Timely
> - Ongoing
> - Consistent

Data from Wiggins, G. (2012). Seven keys to effective feedback. *Educational Leadership, 70*(1). Retrieved from http://www.ascd.org/publications/educational-leadership/sept12/vol70/num01/Seven-Keys-to-Effective-Feedback.aspx.

Constructive feedback needs to be tangible and transparent. Students need to realize how their specific behaviors are affecting their performance. For example, suppose faculty have already discussed the need to check a patient's vital signs every four hours during the clinical day; however, a student continues to forget to take the patient's vital signs at noon. Faculty need to focus on their observation that the student is forgetting to take the noon vital signs and attempt to discover the reasons for this not being done by the student. For example, "Mary, I have noticed you have not taken Mr. Jones's noon vital signs. Please explain to me why Mr. Jones's vital signs were not taken a noon." Perhaps Mary was not aware vital signs needed to be done at noon. At this point, faculty would repeat the clinical expectations related to vital signs monitoring. As faculty, you expect that once students are made aware of their responsibilities, all future nursing care rendered to patients will adhere to these expectations.

Constructive feedback needs to be actionable and focus on the behavior, not the student. Faculty need to be concrete and specific when describing the behavior in question and offer useful or actionable information to help the student. For example, "John, when you taped Mr. Smith's abdominal dressing, the tape was applied over the dressing. Instead, the tape should be applied along the edges of the dressing." Notice that reference is made to how the tape was applied and not to what John did incorrectly. By focusing on the behavior and not on the student's error, you may reduce the student's need to respond defensively.

Constructive feedback needs to be user-friendly and not overload students with too much information they cannot understand. Too much feedback at one time is overwhelming for students and can be counterproductive; therefore, during a feedback session faculty should focus on only one or two important points they want to discuss. The feedback you provide should address the positive as well as the negative behaviors you are noticing from the students. This may help create the learning environment needed to help students feel you are trying to facilitate their learning and improve their performance.

Constructive feedback needs to be timely rather than immediate. In the clinical setting, feedback should be immediate only if students' behaviors are going to compromise patient safety. In most situations, student feedback needs to be provided as soon as possible after the key performance was observed by the faculty. For example, when students complete morning care on their patients and you judge their care as meeting the expectations for patients' hygiene needs, you would provide positive feedback about the care they delivered. If certain students forgot to attend to all patient hygiene needs, however, you would have discussions with these students to elicit their perceptions about the morning care they delivered while providing feedback about the unmet needs of their patients. This discussion and feedback would be done on the same day you made the observations. Providing timely feedback gives students the opportunity to use this feedback to correct their limitations in future situations.

Constructive feedback needs to be ongoing and consistent. This allows students the opportunity to adjust their performance and improve it if it is less than optimal. The more feedback you provide your students that is consistent, reliable, and accurate, the more it may help them improve their clinical performance and satisfy clinical objectives. However, despite your efforts at providing consistent feedback, on some occasions students' performances may fail to meet clinical objectives. In such situations, formative evaluation has not helped improve students' performances, and faculty will need to take this into consideration when completing their summative evaluations.

HOW TO GIVE CONSTRUCTIVE FEEDBACK

As new faculty, you may have a clinical situation that requires you to give constructive feedback to a student. Giving constructive feedback to students who are meeting expectations is, of course, easier than giving constructive feedback to students who are falling below expectations. In either situation, there are some helpful steps you may want to remember.

Step 1: State the purpose for the meeting, why it is important, and what you would like to cover. You may begin the discussion by stating, "I have a concern about the morning care you provided to Mr. Jones" or "I want to discuss your participation in clinical conference." These statements give the student a clear understanding of the topic to be discussed.

Step 2: Describe specifically what you observed the student doing. This should include when and where it happened, who was involved, and what the outcome was. For example, "Yesterday in clinical conference I noticed you were using your smartphone and did not offer a response to the question John asked" or "This morning while you were caring for Mr. Jones, I noticed you did not check his pulse oximeter when he became short of breath."

Step 3: Describe your reaction to the student's behavior. Students need to be told what you have observed about their clinical performance and the possible outcomes of their behavior. You may begin by saying, "I have noticed reluctance on your part to begin morning care on Mr. Jones without getting direction from me. There is the expectation that you will initiate morning care unless you have questions. Waiting for me to give you directions is not acceptable."

Step 4: Give the student an opportunity to respond. Using the example in Step 3, remain silent and wait for a response from the student. If the student hesitates to respond, ask an open-ended question such as "What caused you to hesitate?", "Tell me about this reluctance," or "What do you think about your behavior?"

Step 5: Offer specific suggestions about what the student needs to do to improve the situation. For example, if the student did not position a patient correctly in bed because the patient was weak with limited mobility, you may address the issue by saying, "Rather than leaving the patient in poor body alignment, you can come to me for assistance." This may help the student realize the importance of comfort for the patient and your willingness to help the student in a difficult situation.

Step 6: Summarize your discussion and express your support for helping students meet the clinical objectives. After a discussion with a student, you need to summarize the major points discussed including both positive and negative behaviors. When negative behaviors are discussed, stress the main things the student can do differently to improve performance. Try to end on a positive note by communicating your confidence in the student's ability to improve. By summarizing the student's clinical behaviors, misunderstandings can be avoided and you have an opportunity to show your support for the student's success in the clinical environment.

TIPS FOR CLINICAL EVALUATION

Bonnel (2016) has identified several tips to help faculty responsible for the clinical evaluation process (**Box 10-2**). These tips may help nursing faculty who are new to their roles as clinical instructors to meet the challenges they encounter in evaluating students' clinical competencies fairly and free from biases.

During the clinical orientation, faculty need to review with students the expectations for their performance in the clinical setting. Students need to be informed about what they need to know, the skills they may be required to perform, and the safety precautions needed at all times when delivering patient care. Students will also be expected to transfer the knowledge learned in the classroom to specific patient situations. Informing students of their responsibilities at the beginning of the clinical rotation sets the tone for students to know what is expected from them and how they will be evaluated. You should also review with students the clinical evaluation form and the grading

Box 10-2 Tips for Clinical Evaluation

- Define the knowledge and skills students need to demonstrate during the clinical rotation.
- Use multiple sources of data collection.
- Be reasonable and consistent when evaluating students.
- Use ongoing formative evaluation as a resource to improve student performance.
- Feedback and evaluation should be nonjudgmental and focus on student behaviors.
- When providing evaluation, start with students' strengths and then go to weaknesses.
- Maintain anecdotal records about student behaviors in the clinical setting. Maintain the privacy of this information.
- Make specific notes about students' positive and negative behaviors.
- Document student patterns of behavior over their time spent in the clinical setting.
- Invite students to complete self-assessments summarizing what they have learned.
- Help students prioritize learning needs and set specific goals for each day.

Reproduced from Billings, D. M., & Halstead, J. A. (2016). Clinical performance evaluation. In *Teaching in nursing: A guide for faculty* (5th ed.). St. Louis, MO: Elsevier/Saunders.

criteria used by the school of nursing to determine students' final grades in the clinical rotation.

To evaluate students fairly and consistently, faculty need to use multiple sources of data about students' performances throughout the clinical rotation. A variety of sources should be incorporated into the clinical evaluation to avoid the potential for the evaluation to be subjective and inconsistent. Collecting data from various sources provides faculty with objective and measureable information about students' overall cognitive, psychomotor, and affective abilities. The multiple forms of data collection available to faculty for clinical evaluations will be covered later in this chapter.

Throughout the clinical rotation, faculty need to keep anecdotal notes about their interactions with students and students' reactions to these interactions. Anecdotal notes are defined as "a dated, student-specific notation by a clinical nursing faculty member, describing any component of the student's clinical performance" (Hall, Daly, & Madigan, 2010, p. 157). This note keeping and documentation needs to continue throughout the clinical rotation and may reveal trends in students' level of performance. For example, you may notice from reviewing your notes that a student's performance in the beginning of the clinical rotation was weak and the student required constant assistance from you to ensure the skill was done correctly and safely. However, as the clinical experience continued, the student required less supervision to deliver care safely. Although this student started the clinical rotation with negative-like behaviors, the student's performance improved. Here is another example: If you were assisting a student with a procedure to ensure safety was maintained, how did the student react to your assistance? Did the student willingly accept your assistance, or did the student defend his or her reasons for doing the procedure differently? In both these situations you should realize differences in students' behaviors during the learning process. Therefore, the anecdotal notes you keep on student performance need to include both their positive and negative behaviors.

The evaluation process itself needs to be reasonable, fair, and consistent. This means you need to have the same expectations for all your students when involved in similar situations. It also means you need to take into consideration your expectations of students depending on their level in the nursing program. For example, if you are part of the clinical faculty for freshman nursing students, you should not expect them to be able to prioritize and organize their delivery of nursing care as well as students who are in their senior year. It also means you examine your standards of practice. If safety is an expectation, then any student who does a procedure and violates safety standards should be judged the same.

You need to use ongoing formative evaluation to help improve student performance. Although this is done throughout the clinical rotation, usually midway through the rotation faculty should have a meeting with students to discuss and document their progress. This discussion should be nonjudgmental and focus on their behaviors. You should start with students' positive behaviors and then proceed to the negative ones. This midway evaluation should be the time when students set future goals, make a plan for what they need to do to meet clinical objectives, and identify how they will meet their goals. Faculty need to document the events of this mid-rotation formative evaluation on the clinical evaluation form used by the school of nursing. Because formative evaluation has been linked to guiding and summative evaluation linked to grading, faculty need to do both formative and summative evaluations on students' performances when judging their ability to satisfy clinical objectives and core competencies (Oermann et al., 2009).

DATA COLLECTION METHODS FOR CLINICAL EVALUATION

The goal of clinical evaluation is to form an objective decision about students' ability to satisfy clinical objectives. For this decision to be objective, data about students' cognitive, psychomotor, and affective qualities need to be collected from various resources by various methods. Bonnel (2009) divides these methods into categories and provides some examples of the resources that may be used by faculty to collect data (see **Table 10-1**).

TABLE 10-1 Evaluation Methods and Resources

Method	Resources
Observation	Anecdotal notes
	Checklists
	Rating scales
Written	Charting
	Concept maps
	Nursing care plans
	Process recordings
	Paper and pencil tests
Oral	Student presentations
	Participation in clinical conference discussions
Simulations	Interactive patient simulators
	Role playing and clinical scenarios
Self-evaluation	Clinical portfolio
	Journals and logs

Modified from Bonnel, W. (2016). Clinical performance evaluation. In D. Billings & J. A. Halstead (Eds.), *Teaching in nursing: A guide for faculty* (5th ed., pp. 449–464). St Louis, MO: Elsevier/Saunders.

When faculty plan student evaluations for a clinical course, they need to review the clinical objectives and core competencies before deciding on the methods to use for evaluation. Do the objectives relate to students' achievements in clinical performance, problem solving, critical thinking, or communication? Because evaluating students' performances in the clinical setting is a complex process, it requires the use of more than one resource to judge if the student has met the specific clinical objectives. For example, if the objective was related to students' ability to think critically in the clinical setting, faculty observation, completion of a concept map, and presentation of a case scenario may be the resources faculty use to judge students' ability to meet the objective. Faculty need to decide about the resources they will use to collect data about students' clinical performance. Using various resources for data collection increases the objectivity of the final grade assigned by faculty.

Faculty observation of students in the clinical setting is one way for faculty to evaluation clinical performance (O'Connor, 2015). When observing students, faculty need to consider the contextual aspects of the situation, such as the complexity of the patient care, unexpected environmental events that may interfere with students' abilities to complete assignments, the degree of caring shown to patients during student–patient interactions, the accuracy of student assessments, and the care given to patients, as well as patients' responses to the care they received from students. The data faculty obtain during observation need to be recorded in student-specific anecdotal notes and used later to evaluate students' abilities to meet clinical objectives or core competencies. These written notes serve as part of formative evaluation because they establish a pattern of student behaviors throughout the clinical rotation and can be used later to document students' overall summative evaluation of their clinical performance. When keeping anecdotal notes about student performances, data kept by faculty need to include information about the patients, their needs, and the nursing care administered by the students (see **Box 10-3**).

A sample anecdotal note may be written as follows:

> John was assigned to patient P.T., a 76-year-old male with CHF and COPD. This patient was to receive nebulizer treatments for wheezing and pulse oximeter less than 92%. Student auscultated the lungs and heard wheezing, took the pulse oximeter and results were 91%. Student notified primary nurse to call for respiratory treatment.

This anecdotal note supports the student's ability to deliver care safely and meet clinical objectives. In contrast, if the student did not auscultate the lungs, check the pulse oximeter, and notify the nurse, the evaluation of this student's ability to administer safe nursing care would be judged by faculty as unsatisfactory. In either situation, faculty would provide the necessary feedback to each student; the first student would receive positive feedback, whereas the second student would be informed about behaviors expected in the future to ensure delivery of safe nursing care. Although faculty observations are subjective in nature, anecdotal notes, when written this way, are free from value judgments and state the facts as they occurred. Throughout the clinical rotation, faculty need to keep anecdotal notes on the positive and negatives behaviors they observed with each student to adequately assess each student's performance.

Box 10-3 Data to Include in Anecdotal Notes

- The name of the student who is being evaluated
- The initials of the patient assigned to the student
- Information about the patient's condition, such as medical diagnosis and a brief description of the treatments the patient required during the observation
- A brief description of what the student did or failed to do in providing the necessary care to this patient
- Any factors in the environment or student's behaviors that may have prevented the patient from receiving the necessary care

When observing students' performances, faculty may also use skill checklists and rating scales. A skill checklist often lists the steps to be followed when performing a procedure or skill and is primarily used in the college laboratory. It provides clear instructions to students on how they need to perform a selected skill and can be used as an evaluation tool to verify if students have the beginning abilities to perform the skills. Faculty can use skill checklists to validate students' performances in doing specific skills. Although students may successfully perform the skill on a manikin in the school laboratory, this is not a guarantee they can perform the skill in the clinical setting on a real, live patient. Students have been validated on skills in the laboratory, so they should be able to transfer this learning to the bedside; however, some students may have difficulty doing this and require coaching from you to help them perform the skill correctly. It takes repeated experience doing the skill for students to gain the competence they need to perform it correctly. For this reason, when you assign patients to students, you need to choose patients who have nursing care needs that will help students improve their performance skills.

Rating scales, also referred to as clinical evaluation tools, provide a means of recording faculty judgments about students' observed performances in the clinical setting. These rating scales have two parts: a list of competencies or behaviors students are expected to demonstrate in clinical practice and a scale for rating their performance. There are many rating scales used for evaluating clinical performance, such as pass or fail and satisfactory or unsatisfactory, in addition to multiple-level numerical scales ranging from 1 to 5 points with descriptors. These descriptors may be frequency labels, such as always, usually, frequently, sometimes, or never, or qualitative labels, such as superior, above average, average, or below average. Using rating scales may cause confusion among faculty when they try to determine the differences between above average or average and between a 2 or 1 performance rating. Faculty use of frequency labels may also pose problems because the use of labels requires students to have frequent opportunities to practice and demonstrate the same skill, which we know can be an impossibility given the changing nature of the clinical environment (Gaberson & Oermann, 2015). Although rating scales provide faculty with a convenient form on which to record their judgment of students' clinical performances, faculty need to reach agreement on the type of scale to use and definitions of the descriptors. In addition, faculty cannot lose sight of the biases that may influence their ratings of students and the lack of agreement on the clinical competencies needed by students entering the nursing profession. Regardless of the rating scale faculty choose for their clinical evaluation, this tool should include the behaviors expected from students to meet the course objectives or core competencies defined by the nursing program.

Students' written work also needs to be included in the evaluation process. This written work can reveal students' intellectual abilities to integrate the written work with the clinical assignment. This written work is also an opportunity for faculty to provide formative evaluation that can enhance students' future insights regarding clinical practice. Nursing care plans, concept mappings, and process recordings are some examples of written work that faculty may use to evaluate students' abilities to translate what they have learned in the classroom to real-life situations in the clinical setting. This work can help students organize their thoughts, learn new information, and expand their cognitive abilities. A scoring tool such as a rubric should be developed for use when grading these written assignments to promote consistency and efficiency in grading. Faculty need to decide how these written assignments will be graded—that is, satisfactory, unsatisfactory, or a numerical grade. After faculty review, provide constructive feedback, and grade these assignments, students should be given the opportunity to improve their grade, if needed. This is what it means for faculty to do formative evaluation and provide students with opportunities to improve their summative evaluation.

Oral presentations by students should also be included in the evaluation process. These include case presentations and student participation in clinical conferences. These oral presentations give faculty the opportunity to evaluate students' abilities to express important information in a clear, knowledgeable, organized, and comprehensible manner. Case presentations by students also allow faculty to ask higher-order questions to elicit students' ability to think critically about patient situations and how they would establish priorities for meeting these needs. Discussions in clinical conferences encourage critical thinking among students and allow faculty to focus on the group's ability to problem solve. During clinical conferences, faculty become aware of those students who are more willing to actively participate and offer valuable insight to the discussions. Students' participation in these oral presentations and clinical conferences may contribute to students' achievement of the clinical objectives and core competencies and should be documented on their anecdotal notes.

Gaberson and Oermann (2015) present criteria that faculty need to use when evaluating clinical conferences. These include the ability of students to do the following:

- Present ideas clearly and in a logical, organized way
- Participate actively in group discussions
- Offer ideas relevant to the topic being discussed
- Demonstrate knowledge of the topic
- Offer different perspectives on the topic to encourage critical thinking among group members
- Assume a leadership role in facilitating group discussions and problem solving

If your nursing program uses simulations for clinical experience, these sessions may also be included in the evaluation process. The case studies used in simulations provide students with the semi-realistic experiences they may be exposed to in the clinical setting. Students are expected to respond to these situations by conducting assessments, identifying patient needs, carrying out interventions, and evaluating the outcomes of their interventions. Simulation provides students with the opportunity to apply the steps in the nursing process while making decisions and evaluating the effectiveness of their decisions. Students' actions during the simulation give faculty insight into students' abilities to administer knowledgeable, safe care; to think critically; and to problem solve and make decisions. In most situations, simulation is used as formative evaluation, but it may also be used for summative evaluation. If faculty decide to include simulation in the evaluation process, they need to decide which clinical objectives or competencies will be judged using simulation and whether simulation will be used for grading purposes. If used for grading purposes in summative evaluation, faculty need to develop checklists for rating students' performances.

Self-evaluation is another method that helps students consider their progress in clinical learning. Self-evaluation needs to begin in the first clinical course and continue throughout the program. Self-evaluations are usually completed midway through the clinical course and give students the opportunity to assess their own clinical performances and identify their strengths and areas for improvement. Discussions with students about their self-evaluations and perceptions of their performances provide faculty with opportunities to structure feedback and identify areas where students need to improve. Using students' own assessments, faculty can develop plans for helping students improve their practice in situations that pose problems and guide them on methods to improve critical-thinking, problem-solving, and decision-making skills.

Clinical portfolios and students' journals or logs are additional methods faculty can implement in a clinical course to help monitor students' progress. Portfolios are a collection of students' work throughout the course or curriculum and can be used to assess students' progress toward achievement of clinical objectives or core competencies. Portfolios may be used in undergraduate and graduate nursing programs. When portfolios are used in nursing programs, faculty need to establish guidelines for compiling and evaluating the content of these portfolios.

Students' journals or logs enable students to express their thoughts about their clinical experiences in written form. Students make weekly entries into their logs about what they experienced in the clinical setting, what they may have learned from these experiences, and their reactions to this learning experience. Through journaling, students have an opportunity to reflect on their learning experiences, work logically through the process, and, one hopes, gain insight into their own self-awareness. The journal should include a description of each event, an analysis by students of how they handled the experiences, and self-reflections that identify students' strengths, weaknesses, and areas for improvement (Billings & Halstead, 2012). Faculty need to maintain the confidentiality of student journals and provide feedback about students' efforts, not feedback about the student as an individual. Faculty feedback on students' journal entries is an important part of the teaching/learning process and requires a trusting relationship between student and faculty.

WORKING WITH PROBLEM STUDENTS IN THE CLINICAL SETTING

Faculty would like to believe that all students assigned to them for a clinical rotation will be safe, knowledgeable, and competent individuals. Unfortunately, this is not the case. Some students will be stellar in their performance, whereas others will lag behind. It is important for faculty to identify students with limited clinical abilities early in the clinical rotation so you can offer them the help they need to improve their clinical performance.

Zuzelo (2000) offers some suggestions for helping students at risk. First, criteria for student success should be understood by all students. Students who are at risk need to know how their behaviors are not meeting clinical objectives, and faculty need to document these patterns of marginal behaviors. This information is documented by faculty in anecdotal notes and shared with the student at the time of the observation or at the formative evaluation meeting. Also at this time, a remedial plan is put together by faculty and students to help these students at risk improve their clinical performance. Next, a written contract of this remedial plan is developed and signed by the students at risk and the faculty. This written contract clearly identifies faculty's and students' responsibilities for satisfying this performance improvement plan.

Any conferences faculty have with at-risk students should be held in a quiet, private area. A written summary of the discussion should be prepared that includes the date, time, who was present, clinical performance issues, outcome plans, and time frame for completion. This written documentation is signed by students and faculty and is part of students' formative evaluations. Faculty observations and documentation should not be limited to only students at risk. Faculty need to plan for performance observations of each student and avoid focusing on only students who are at risk for failure. Doing this may leave some students at risk of feeling victimized; however, some students who are marginal and receive feedback to improve their performance do not object to this extra attention (Gaberson & Oermann, 2015).

Faculty need to adhere to the nursing program's policies on clinical performance. At times, if students' clinical behaviors are potentially unsafe, faculty may be required to remove students from the clinical setting and send them for remedial help in the college laboratory. At other times, faculty may need to provide constructive feedback to students about their unsafe performances and share with them the expected behaviors required to pass the course. In any case, all students have the right to know how they are performing throughout the clinical rotation. More importantly, students at risk have the right to know what they need to do to improve their clinical performance and the consequences of their continuing failure to meet course expectations. This is known as due process, and faculty should adhere to this before deciding to assign failing grades to students for their clinical performances.

Once at-risk students have been made aware of how their marginal performance is not meeting clinical objectives and what they need to do to improve their clinical performance, faculty should provide these students with repeated experiences that offer opportunities for them to improve. However, if repeated attempts by at-risk students to improve their clinical performance have been unsuccessful, faculty need to consider failing these students for this clinical rotation. Nursing programs have written policies about failures in classroom and clinical courses. In some programs students may be allowed to repeat one nursing course before being dismissed from the program. When you accept a job as a clinical instructor, you must be familiar with the nursing program's provisions for due process as well as policies concerning grading, progression in the program, graduation, and dismissal. You also need to be familiar with the college's policy on grade appeal.

GRADING CLINICAL PRACTICE: THE GOOD, THE BAD, AND THE UGLY

At the end of a clinical rotation, faculty are required to assign a clinical grade for each student. The type of clinical grade assigned will be determined by nursing department policy. In most schools of nursing, guidelines for the course grading indicate that students must pass the clinical component to pass the course. In other situations, separate grading may be given for classroom theory and clinical practice.

Assigning grades to students' clinical performances is neither an easy task nor a decision easily made. Unlike grading written examinations that measure students' performances objectively, faculty use subjective data observed throughout the clinical rotation to decide students' final clinical performance grades. When deciding on students' clinical grades, faculty need to take into consideration whether students' clinical performances have demonstrated progressive improvement toward attainment of agreed-upon course objectives or clinical competencies. The multiple sources of data collection used by faculty during the clinical rotation and their results provide faculty with the information needed to make this important decision. These data results should be grouped according to course objectives or competencies so faculty can judge whether students have met the outcomes for the course. If these evaluation methods were given a numerical value, these grades can be incorporated into the overall clinical evaluation. After reviewing the data collected on all students' performances, faculty should be able to assign students their clinical grades.

To help faculty arrive at students' final clinical grades, O'Conner (2015) encourages faculty to seek answers to the following questions:

- Has the student demonstrated at least a minimal level of competence in meeting course objectives and core competencies?

- Did the student demonstrate growth and development in his or her knowledge of patient care needs and ability to perform skills safely with less directed assistance from the instructor?
- Did the student demonstrate increasing confidence in assuming responsibility for patient care?
- Has the student demonstrated the knowledge and skills necessary to move forward to the next level in the nursing program?
- Was the student's practice safe throughout the clinical rotation?

Responses to these questions will help faculty decide whether students should pass or fail the clinical course. To help answer these questions, faculty need to review the data collected on students' performances throughout the clinical rotation and their formative evaluations. Affirmative answers to these questions support a passing grade, whereas negative responses substantiate students' failure to meet course objectives and faculty's decision to assign a failing grade.

In addition to assigning a grade for clinical evaluation, faculty should write on the evaluation tool a description of each student's overall performance in relation to his or her achievement of clinical objectives. This information provides students with feedback that is more useful to them than a simple grade and lets them know how they are developing toward their goal of entering the nursing profession. For those students who did not pass the clinical rotation, this written evaluation provides feedback to them about their future possibilities for progression in the nursing program and their entry into the nursing profession.

At times faculty have difficulty assigning a failing clinical grade to a student because they are concerned about the legal ramifications of their decision. Any lawsuits filed against nursing programs and nursing faculty due to students' clinical failures have ruled in favor of the nursing program and faculty, as long as the institution followed administrative policies and procedures and the decision was viewed as fair, rather than arbitrary or discriminatory (Westrick, 2007). Therefore, to avoid charges of discriminatory practices, faculty need to keep scrupulous records on students' performance throughout the clinical rotation and the extra assistance they provided to help at-risk students improve. The remediation provided to at-risk students should be ongoing throughout the rotation and documented at mid-semester at the time of the formative evaluation. Students need to be kept aware of their progress toward achieving clinical objectives and informed about the consequences if their performance does not improve by the end of the clinical rotation. Nursing program administration should be kept informed about impending clinical performance problems early in the rotation because their support is essential when performance is determined to be unsatisfactory.

If faculty decide a student should receive a failing clinical grade, both the student and administration should be notified immediately. Failing students may react in several different ways. They may respond with denial by making excuses for how specific events occurred or did not occur. They may seek to blame the instructor for not being available to help them. They may even accuse the instructor of being discriminatory and "out to get them." Faculty need to stand firm with their decision and remain focused on the events that occurred throughout the clinical rotation that contributed to the student's final evaluation and the decision made. Students have the right to respond to their failing grade and should be informed about the college's grade appeal process if they intend to seek additional help with this decision.

SUMMARY

Clinical evaluation of nursing students is a challenging responsibility for nursing faculty. This chapter explored the process of clinical evaluation and those challenges faculty encounter when judging students' performance in the clinical setting. The reliability of these judgments is supported by the various data collection methods faculty use throughout the clinical rotation. Clinical objectives and core competencies need to be the framework used for judging students' ability to deliver safe care to their assigned patients. Clinical evaluation provides both subjective and objective data for formative and summative evaluation. Assigning a grade to students' clinical performance requires faculty to respond to critical questions about students' behaviors and relationships with their patients. Responses to these questions may require faculty to judge some students in ways that prevent them from moving forward in the nursing program.

CASE STUDIES

1. You are the clinical faculty for a group of eight freshman nursing students who will spend a 15-week clinical rotation on a medical–surgical unit in an acute care hospital. Last week was the first day of this rotation, and time was spent providing these students with a general orientation to the unit and introduction to the nursing staff. The clinical objectives, core competencies, and evaluation tool were reviewed with the students on the first day. Clinical assignments with due dates were explained to the students. Discussions about student and faculty expectations during this rotation were also shared.

   On week 2 of this rotation, a student was assigned a patient who required dressing changes once a day. This was the student's first time doing dressing changes for a real, live patient situation, so you asked the student to seek your assistance before doing the dressing change.

At the end of the clinical day you observed the patient's dressing had not been changed.

   a. How would you handle this situation?

   b. What action would you expect from the student?

   c. What feedback would you provide to the student?

   d. How would you provide this constructive feedback to the student?

   e. How you would document the event?

   f. How would you handle your future observations of this student's clinical performance?

2. Your 15-week clinical rotation with the students is in the 12th week and due to end soon. The clinical performance of one student has not been meeting course objectives. You met with this student at week 8, completed a formative evaluation, and together developed an improvement plan. The time to make your final decision about this student's clinical grade is quickly approaching.

   a. Which data would you use to help you make your final decision?

   b. When reviewing these data, which questions might you ask yourself while judging this student's ongoing performance?

   c. What are your faculty responsibilities when a student is at risk for failing a clinical course?

   d. How would you document your evaluation and communicate your final decision to this student?

REFERENCES

Benner, P. (1982). *From novice to expert: Excellence to power in clinical nursing practice.* Menlo Park, CA: Addison Wesley.

Bonnel, W. (2016). Clinical performance evaluation. In D. Billings & J. A. Halstead (Eds.), *Teaching in nursing: A guide for faculty* (5th ed., pp. 449–464). St. Louis, MO: Elsevier/Saunders.

Bransford, J. D., Brown, A. L., & Cocking, R. R. (Eds.). (2000). *How people learn: Brain, mind experience, and school.* Washington, DC: National Academy Press.

Dean, C. B., Hubbell, E. R., Pitler, H., & Stone, B. J. (2012). *Classroom instruction that works: Research based strategies for increasing student achievement.* Alexandria, VA: Association for Supervision and Curriculum.

Edmond, C. B. (2001). A new paradigm for practice education. *Nurse Education Today, 21,* 251–259.

Gaberson, K. B., & Oermann, M. H. (2015). *Clinical teaching strategies in nursing* (4th ed.). New York, NY: Springer.

Hall, M. A., Daley, B. J., & Madigan, E. A. (2010). Use of anecdotal notes by clinical nursing faculty: A descriptive study. *Journal of Nursing Education, 49*(3), 156–159.

Hattie, J. (2008). *Visible learning: A synthesis of over 800 meta-analyses relating to achievement.* New York, NY: Routledge.

Holaday, S. D., & Buckley, K. M. (2008). A standardized clinical evaluation tool-kit: Improving nursing education and practice. *Annual Review of Nursing Education, 6,* 123–149.

Karayurt, O., Mert, H., & Beser, A. (2008). A study on the development of a scale to assess nursing students' performance in the clinical setting. *Journal of Clinical Nursing, 18*, 1123–1130.

Mahara, M. S. (1998). A perspective on clinical evaluation in nursing education. *Journal of Advanced Nursing, 28*(6), 1339–1346.

O'Conner, A. B. (2015). *Clinical instruction and evaluation: A faculty resource* (3rd ed.). Burlington, MA: Jones & Bartlett Learning.

Oermann, M. H., & Gaberson, K. (2014). *Evaluation and testing in nursing education* (4th ed.). New York, NY: Springer.

Oermann, M. H., Yarbough, S. S., Saewert, K. J., Ard, N., & Charasika, M. (2009). Clinical evaluation and grading practices in schools of nursing. *Nursing Education Perspectives, 30*(6), 352–357.

Parra, M. R., Guerrero, A. G., Mayor, S. G., Uttumchandani, S. K., Campos, A. L., & Asencio, J. M. M. (2015). Design of a competency evaluation model for clinical nursing practicum based on standardized language systems: Psychometric validation study. *Journal of Nursing Scholarship, 47*(4), 371–376.

Reising, D. L., & Devich, L. E. (2004). Comprehensive practicum evaluation across a nursing program. *Nursing Education Perspectives, 25*(3), 114–119.

Scriven, M. (1991). *Evaluation thesaurus* (4th ed.). Newbury Park, CA: Sage.

Skingley, A., Arnott, J., Graves, J., & Nabb, J. (2006). Supporting practice teachers to identify failing students. *British Journal of Community Nursing, 12*(1), 28–32.

Sroczyznski, M., Gravil, G., Route, P. S., Hoffart, N., & Creelmann, P. (2011). Creativity and connections: The future of nursing education and practice: The Massachusetts initiative. *Journal of Professional Nursing* [online], *27*(6), e64–e70.

Walsh, T., Jairath, N., Paterson, M. A., & Grandjean, C. (2010). Quality and safety for nurses clinical evaluation tool. *Journal of Nursing Education, 49*(9), 517–522.

Westrick, S. J. (2007). Legal challenges to academic decisions. *Journal of Nursing Law, 11*(2), 104–107.

Wiggins, G. (2012). Seven keys to effective feedback. *Educational Leadership, 70*(1), 10–16. Retrieved from http://www.ascd.org/publications/educational-leadership/sept12/vol70/num01/Seven-Keys-to-Effective-Feedback.aspx

Zuzelo, P. R. (2000). Clinical issues, clinical probation: Supporting the at-risk student. *Nurse Educator, 25*(5), 216–218.

CHAPTER 11

Legal Issues in Clinical Nursing Education

OBJECTIVES

- Explain due process and its application in clinical nursing education.
- Explain the standard for patient care and how it applies to faculty and students in the clinical setting.
- Recognize safe and unsafe clinical practices among nursing students.
- Examine the common areas of negligence and liability for nurse educators and understand how they influence your responsibilities in the clinical setting.
- Differentiate faculty responsibilities and actions in the clinical setting that may limit your liability for negligence.

The nursing profession is regulated by federal, state, and local laws that have implications for our practice. One well-known practice law developed by the State Board of Nursing in each state is the state's Nurse Practice Act. These state-specific acts define the nursing profession's scope of practice when administering nursing care to patients. As practicing nurses, we adhere to these state regulations because we know that if we practice outside these regulations we may be liable for negligence in the delivery of care to our patients. There are also policies within our place of employment that define the legal role of the nurse in that agency. Which legal concerns may arise for nurses who have become clinical educators supervising the administration of nursing care by students?

This chapter will explore the legal rights and duties of faculty and students involved in clinical teaching situations and offer suggestions for preventing, minimizing, and managing difficult situations that may pose a liability for negligence by the parties involved. However, it is beyond the scope of this text to interpret the law because the authors are not qualified to give any legal advice to clinical educators regarding their practice. Clinical educators need to refer questions about their legal right to practice as educators to the legal counsel at their place of employment.

The legal concept of due process law is placed at the beginning of this chapter because it is the fundamental principle of fairness in regard to the rights of each individual in all legal matters. The aim of due process is to safeguard these public and private rights against unfairness. As a clinical educator you need to understand this legal process because it will be used by the courts in deciding your rights and those of your students and the patients they care for in clinical teaching situations.

DUE PROCESS

Due process is a constitutional guarantee found in the Fifth and Fourteenth Amendments to the U.S. Constitution that prohibits all levels of government from arbitrarily or unfairly depriving individuals of their basic constitutional rights to life, liberty, and property (The Free Dictionary, n.d.). In higher education, due process refers to the provision of a fair and just opportunity for students to explain and defend their actions against charges of misconduct or to challenge decisions made by colleges or universities related to program admission, retention, suspension, dismissal, or final course grades (Southeastern Oklahoma State University, n.d.). Hopefully, given this brief explanation of due process for individuals, including patients, and students in higher education, you may begin to understand how the right to due process can impact your role as an educator in the clinical setting.

The application of constitutional due process is divided into two categories: substantive due process and procedural due process. Substantive due process law creates, defines, and regulates individuals' rights, whereas procedural due process law enforces those rights or seeks amends for their violation. Substantive due process is viewed as an academic due process by the courts when due process law is applied to education. To ensure academic due process is adhered to in institutions of higher learning, the following procedures are generally sufficient (Gaberson & Oermann, 2015):

- Students are informed in advance of the academic standards that will be used to judge their performance.
- Students are notified about the potential for academic failure well before any final grading decisions are made. This notification is done orally and put in writing, and together the teacher and the student develop a plan for overcoming any deficiencies.
- Students' performances are evaluated using the stated standards, and grades are assigned according to the stated policy.
- When students believe a grade or other academic decision is unfair, the institution's grade appeal or grievance process is followed. Usually the first step is for students to discuss the grade appeal with the teacher. If the appeal is not resolved at this level, students have the right to appeal to the administrator to whom the teacher reports. The next level of appeal may be to a specialized panel of decision makers defined by the institution's policy. Finally, students should have the right to appeal the decision to the highest-level academic administrator in the institution.

- If students are not satisfied with the institution's decision, they have the right to seek a decision from the courts. The courts will allow such a lawsuit to move forward only if the students have exhausted all internal institutional remedies.

Clinical educators need to be very cognizant of these procedures to ensure due process law has been followed when implementing their roles as clinical educators. Your knowledge and understanding of these procedures should guide your interactions with students in the clinical setting. If you do not apply these procedures when evaluating your students, you may be held liable in your role as a clinical educator. Conversely, if faculty and administrators have followed these substantive due process procedures, it is unlikely the academic decision will be overturned. The courts traditionally have been reluctant to intervene in academic decisions because they believe faculty are competent to judge student performances according to academic standards (Brent, 2004a). However, this is not to say the courts have not intervened in faculty decisions. Courts have intervened when substantive due process has not been followed, as will be shown later in this chapter. However, when students appeal to courts of law, the burden of proof rests with the students to prove academic due process was denied to them.

Procedural due process is the second category of constitutional due process law that involves disciplinary decisions. Procedural due process is a higher level of due process law that governs how legal proceedings must be carried out and guarantees the right to a notice and hearing before disciplinary decisions are made. In other words, in legal or administrative proceedings, any person or student who might be negatively impacted by the outcome, such as dismissal from an educational program or school, has the right to be told a proceeding is going to take place, has the right to appear before a neutral judge or arbitrator, and has the right to explain his or her side of the case before a decision is made (Rottenstein Law Group, n.d.).

When procedural due process involves a student's dismissal from a program or institution of higher education for misconduct, dishonesty, or academic failure, disciplinary due process needs to include the following components (Gaberson & Oermann, 2015):

- Students are provided with adequate written notice identifying the specific details of their acts of misconduct, dishonesty, or academic failure. However, not all acts of misconduct may require immediate dismissal from an academic program or institution. The institution's dismissal policy should be clearly identified in its policy manual and student handbook.
- Students are provided opportunities for fair, impartial hearings on the charges against them and have the right to speak on their own behalf as well as question the administrators and faculty involved in the case. Both students and faculty are entitled to legal counsel in this situation.

- Students have the right to seek a decision from the courts if they believe procedural due process was not followed. However, once again the burden of proof rests with the student.

While in nursing programs, nursing students are held to the same standard of care as registered nurses. The overall standard for patient care is what an ordinary, reasonable, and prudent nurse would have done in a similar situation. The rationale underlying this standard of care is that patients have the right to expect the professional services delivered by the hospital or healthcare agency to be provided by persons with professional skills and competence (Guido, 2006, p. 504). If clinical actions by students do not satisfy the standard for patient care, a case for professional negligence and liability may exist. Negligence is defined as "the failure to exercise the standard of care that a reasonably prudent person would have exercised in a similar situation" (Davis, 2002, p. 191). In nursing practice, the standard applies to the nursing care delivered by a registered professional nurse. Therefore, faculty and the students they supervise in the clinical setting are expected to deliver the same standard of care to patients that registered nurses employed by the agency would give to their patients. Students are responsible for their own actions as long as they are performing according to the standards set forth by the school of nursing and they seek assistance from faculty when they are uncertain how to deliver their nursing care. For this reason, it is not true that students practice under their faculty's license (Brent, 2004b). Students' right to due process comes into play if faculty determine students' actions in the clinical setting do not satisfy the overall standard for patient care.

Applying Due Process in the Clinical Environment

Faculty are required to adhere to due process when evaluating students in the clinical setting, and their evaluations must ensure fair and just treatment for all clinical students. When determining whether fair and just treatment was given to all students in the clinical setting, the courts will seek to determine whether students received due process from the educational institution. Fairness involves implementation of procedural issues; equity implies that like cases are treated the same unless special circumstances apply; and duties and rights are those responsibilities of the parties involved (Miller, 1996). Table 11-1 identifies these due process concepts and their application in the clinical education environment (Scanlan, 2001).

It is essential for clinical faculty to understand and follow these four due process concepts when evaluating students' clinical performances. To uphold fairness and equity when evaluating students, faculty need to apply the criteria and standards defined by the school of nursing to determine safe clinical performance by students. These criteria and standards need to be consistently applied to all students when evaluating their clinical performance. Adherence to the nursing program's policies regarding faculty

TABLE 11-1 Due Process Concepts in Clinical Education

Due Process Concept	Application in Clinical Education
Fairness	• Examination of evidence • Application of criteria and standards • Clarification of criteria and standards • Documentation of decisions
Equity	• Consistent application of procedures • Alteration of procedures when justified
Duties	Faculty: • Adequate preparation of students • Fair assessment • Maintenance of documentation • Ensuring safe care • Conveying information to students Students: • Providing safe care • Preparing for practice • Knowing personal limitations
Rights	Faculty: • Evaluating students • Determining grades • Removing students from practice when warranted • Questioning professional suitability Students: • Receiving timely feedback • Receiving and reviewing supporting evidence • Receiving timely notice of decisions • Challenging negative data and/or evidence • Being assisted by a person of their choice • Including objections in a permanent record

Reproduced from Scanlan, J. M. (2001). Dealing with the unsafe student in clinical practice. *Nurse Educator,* 26(1), 23–27.

roles and responsibilities in the clinical setting may avoid any legal concerns related to faculty bias or discrimination toward students.

Due process also requires faculty to satisfy certain duties toward students assigned to their clinical rotation. In previous chapters we explored faculty's responsibilities as clinical instructors. Faculty need to provide students with information about agency policies and procedures related to student nurses; an orientation to the clinical facility and introduction to the staff; information about the clinical objectives; expectations for delivering safe nursing care; and course evaluation methods. Faculty duties toward students do not stop here; they continue throughout the clinical rotation. Faculty need to assess students' abilities and delegate patient assignments consistent with the knowledge and skills students have achieved thus far in the nursing program. Faculty need to document students' clinical performance objectively by identifying students' strengths and weaknesses when performing nursing skills. Faculty need to provide students with timely feedback about their clinical performances and be available to help them to improve, if needed. Faculty, together with students, need to develop a corrective plan of action that helps students improve in their future delivery of safe nursing care. Faculty need to provide students with fair assessments of their clinical performance that include data collected from other sources aside from faculty clinical observations. Other sources of data collection that can be used to determine students' competencies in the clinical environment are discussed in Chapter 10.

Students also have duties to perform during their clinical rotations. They must adhere to the nursing program's policies defined in the student handbook as well as any agency policies related to student nurses. Students have a duty to come to the clinical experience prepared for practice and ready to apply the knowledge and skills learned in the classroom to ensure delivery of safe care to their patients in the clinical setting. Students have a duty to know the clinical objectives and the standards by which their nursing care will be evaluated. Students must know their limitations and openly share these limitations with faculty before attempting to deliver care to their assigned patients. Students must ask for help from faculty when they are unsure of their ability to safely meet patients' needs.

Emerson (2007) provides some definitions for safe and unsafe behaviors among students in the clinical setting that may serve as a guide for faculty when evaluating the quality of students' clinical performances (**Box 11-1**).

Academic due process also defines faculty's and students' rights. In the case of clinical education, clinical faculty have the right to evaluate students, determine grades, and remove students from the clinical setting if they are deemed unsafe to practice. Nursing students have the right to receive timely feedback from their clinical instructor about their clinical practice. When students receive unsatisfactory grades in their clinical performance, they have the right to receive timely notice of this decision, review the data supporting this decision, and challenge the evidence with assistance from a person of their choice. Educational institutions that remain compliant with due process law will have a clearly defined process for students to follow when a grade dispute exists. Faculty needs to be aware of the educational institution's policy for student grade appeals.

Specific court cases that help illustrate the application of this provision for due process in higher education will be presented later in this chapter. When you read these

Box 11-1 Definitions of Safe and Unsafe Clinical Practice

Safe Student Clinical Practice
- Students are expected to demonstrate growth in their ability to deliver nursing care through the application of the knowledge and skills learned from courses throughout the nursing program.
- Students' growth in clinical practice needs to meet the clinical expectations outlined in each clinical course evaluation tool.
- Students are expected to be prepared for clinical practice by having the knowledge needed to deliver safe nursing care and by being prepared to carry out the skills necessary to deliver this care to assigned patients. These student expectations are outlined in each course syllabus.

Unsafe Student Clinical Practice
- Unsafe clinical practice is student clinical behavior that places the patient in either physical or emotional jeopardy.
  - Physical jeopardy is the delivery of care to patients that creates a risk of physical harm.
  - Emotional jeopardy occurs when the student creates an environment of anxiety or distress that puts the patient or staff at risk for emotional or psychological harm.
- Unsafe clinical practice is an occurrence or pattern of repeated behaviors that places patients at risk for injury.

Data from Emerson, R. J. (2007). Legal and ethical implications in the clinical education setting. In *Nursing education in the clinical setting* (pp. 86–101). St. Louis, MO: Mosby-Elsevier.

cases you may want to consider the actions of the faculty and students that may have contributed to their liability for negligence. Ideally, after reviewing these cases, you will have better insight into how to avoid these situations in your role as a clinical educator.

LIABILITY FOR NEGLIGENCE BY FACULTY

Faculty are not liable for the negligent acts of their students, provided: (1) they have selected appropriate learning activities based on the course objectives and core competencies; (2) they have determined that students have acquired the course material that provides them with the knowledge, skills, and attitudes necessary to complete their clinical assignments; and (3) they provide guidance throughout the clinical rotation (Gaberson, 2015, p. 102). However, faculty can be held liable for negligence if they make clinical assignments that require more knowledge and skill than students have learned in the classroom or if they fail to provide adequate guidance to their students. For this reason, clinical faculty should carry their own professional liability insurance (O'Conner, 2006, pp. 304, 306).

TABLE 11-2 Common Areas of Negligence and Liability for Nurse Educators

- Failure to properly delegate duties to a student
- Failure to properly document student's nursing skills
- Failure to require students to obtain more education in areas of poor performance
- Failure to adequately notify students of areas of failure or poor performance
- Failure to discuss or present a plan for improvement
- Failure to facilitate student due process
- Failure to protect student safety

Data from Aiken, 2004; Goudreau, 2002. Reproduced from Emerson, R. J. (2007). Legal and ethical implications in the clinical education setting. In *Nursing education in the clinical setting* (pp. 86–101). St. Louis, MO: Mosby-Elsevier.

Emerson (2007) identifies common areas of negligence and liability for nurse educators (**Table 11-2**).

Nursing faculty may be involved in legal actions involving students by being named a codefendant, along with the school or college, or they may be sued individually. In a court of law, legal actions against nurse educators fall under tort law, which is civil law dealing with wrongs committed by one person against another. In addition to a patient suing a student for the care received, the patient may sue the clinical instructor, the educator's school of nursing, and the hospital. Three elements need to exist for the charge of tort to be made against a clinical educator regarding the actions of a student toward a patient: (1) The accused student had a duty or obligation to a patient while under the supervision of the clinical instructor; (2) there was a breach or violation of the duty because the nurse educator failed to meet the standard of care; and (3) the patient must have suffered harm as a result of the breach in the nurse educator's performance of duty (Glasgow, Dreher, & Oxholm, 2012).

Nurse educators and nursing programs can apply several strategies to reduce the risk of lawsuits and decrease nurse educator liability. Clinical teaching assignments need to adhere to Board of Nursing regulations for faculty–student ratios. In the United States this faculty-led clinical ratio is 1:10, and for prelicensure preceptor-led clinical experiences the ratio is 1:1 (Lewallen, DeBrew, & Stump, 2014). Faculty and preceptors should be adequately prepared for their roles through formal education and experience. Nursing faculty should be provided with an orientation by the school of nursing that includes clear and concise information about the course content, student learning outcomes, and core competencies. Faculty should meet with agency staff to learn agency policies, build working relationships, and enhance communication with the nurses on their assigned units. Good relationships with the nurses on the unit may improve the exchange of information among faculty and staff about student performances so that unsafe actions by students can be corrected (Patton& Lewallen, 2015). Faculty should also be aware of the needs of each patient assigned to a nursing student and conduct daily interviews with patients and families regarding the care they received from the students. Faculty who maintain good relationships with patients and families are less likely to have legal actions brought against them (Shipman, 2010).

To further limit legal liability for faculty, students are prepared to administer nursing care in a laboratory setting prior to beginning their clinical rotation in a healthcare agency. In this laboratory setting, students should be validated in their ability to perform basic nursing skills such as handwashing, needle safety, infection control, and lifting/transferring techniques, as well as other nursing skills defined by the nursing program such as suctioning, tube feeding, and Foley catheter insertion. While in the clinical area, the nurse educator should assess students' abilities and limitations and set benchmarks for students before allowing them to progress. At times, students may need to be directed to return to the college laboratory for additional practice before being allowed to perform the skill on a real, live patient. Any concerns about a student's performance should be discussed immediately with the student, and the student should be instructed to seek faculty supervision before delivering nursing care.

Having preclinical and postclinical conferences at the clinical site may also limit liability. These conferences provide opportunities for faculty to discuss students' questions about their patient assignments while assessing their readiness to deliver safe nursing care.

Faculty need to consider the strengths and weaknesses of their students when making clinical assignments. If faculty assign patients to students who do not have the knowledge and skills needed to deliver safe nursing care, they may be held liable for the assignment they made. For this reason, when you are hired as a clinical instructor you need to be familiar with the course syllabus containing the course content and the student learning outcomes.

LIABILITY FOR NEGLIGENCE BY STUDENTS

Nursing students always retain accountability for their own knowledge and the nursing care they deliver during their clinical rotations. Because they are ultimately responsible for their own actions, they may be held liable for their own negligence. Students must be knowledgeable in the content taught throughout the nursing program and be aware of hospital policies and procedures as they relate to implementation by students. Faculty must ensure students understand these hospital policies and procedures, and students are required to adhere to them. If students administer nursing care that exceeds their role as students and patients suffer harm, students are more likely to incur sole responsibility for their actions because they have been informed earlier by faculty of their role as students. Students must be knowledgeable about patients' conditions and physicians' orders for medications and treatments. Students are expected to follow these orders to ensure patient safety. Students who implement nursing care that does not adhere to physicians' orders may be held liable for negligence. Students who are uncertain about their ability to perform a procedure or skill and feel they need additional supervision must ask for help from the clinical instructor. Clinical faculty have a duty to adequately supervise and assist students when needed. If faculty do not help students when needed and fail to prevent unsafe nursing practices by students, faculty as well as students may incur potential liability for negligence (Guido, 2006).

Liability for healthcare agencies, faculty, and students may be decreased by having a contract between the clinical agency and the school of nursing. Healthcare agencies agree to accept a predetermined number of clinical nursing students, and the school of nursing agrees to prescreen the nursing students prior to their coming to the clinical agency. The educational institution must ensure students' academic grades support their competence to practice in a clinical setting under the direct supervision of a qualified clinical instructor. Healthcare agencies must maintain safe clinical sites that meet the standards of care for all patients. Both the educational institution and the clinical agency have an equal duty to each other to ensure a safe environment for students and patients where the standard of care is maintained throughout (Guido, 2006, p. 506).

CASES INVOLVING NEGLIGENCE, LIABILITY, AND MISCONDUCT

This section explores litigation cases involving student and faculty liability for negligence when the standard of care owed to patients is violated. Cases involving students' misconduct in nursing programs and faculty responsibility to respect the due process rights of these students are also presented. Reviewing these cases may help you asses the current levels of risk associated with your employment as a clinical nurse educator.

In clinical education, nursing students and the faculty who supervise them are expected to follow the same standard of care owed to patients by registered nurses employed by the healthcare agency. In the case of *Lovett v. Lorain Community Hospital* (2004), a patient was given an intramuscular injection of Demerol and Vistaril by a nursing student who was under the direct supervision of a clinical instructor. The negligence alleged by the patient was that the injection was given incorrectly, causing permeant damage to the sciatic nerve. The patient sued the student, the instructor, and the hospital. The case proceeded against the nursing student, the instructor, and the hospital. The clinical instructor who supervised the administration of this injection had the responsibility to ensure this student gave the injection correctly (Guido, 2006, p. 204).

In another liability case, *Blanding v. Richland Memorial Hospital* (1988), an 18-year-old patient suffered a cardiac arrest and died following simple skin graft surgery. The nursing student who was taking care of him failed to notice that he had stopped breathing. There was student liability in this case plus liability to the instructor and nursing staff at the institution. Because nursing students remain accountable for their knowledge and skills, faculty and staff may become accountable for individual student incompetence or unpreparedness. To limit faculty liability for student incompetence, faculty need to clearly communicate clinical expectations to students at the beginning of the rotation, properly supervise the student throughout the clinical experience, and remove any students from the clinical site who have demonstrated unsafe practice.

Unlike in the *Blanding* case, in *Dimora v. Cleveland Clinic Foundation* (1996) liability was limited to the nursing student. An elderly patient was harmed because the nursing student failed to ensure the patient's safety. The patient had fallen backward several times in the past, and her medical chart clearly indicated that she had serious difficulties with balance and needed assistance when standing and walking. The nursing student had read the patient's chart, but nonetheless when helping the patient up from the toilet, the student left the patient standing alone with her walker and walked away to open the door. The patient fell backward and was injured. An expert witness testified that a nursing student at this level should have been able to safely care for this patient. The student testified she had received training to assist patients with ambulation and transfer while in the nursing program and had passed those skills. Liability in this case was assessed against the student (Guido, 2006, p. 205).

Faculty and students are also charged with following hospital policy, and faculty have a duty to allow only competent students the right to practice in clinical settings. In the case of *Humpert v. Bay Medical Center* (2003), an elderly patient was admitted for surgery to place a shunt to drain cranial fluid. Following surgery, the patient was confused and required physical restraints, and a bed sensor alarm was placed on the patient's bed. Neither the restraints nor the bed alarm was in use when the patient fell out of bed. The patient fractured her hip, was returned to surgery, and later died of complications. In the trial that ensued, one of the main issues concerned the nursing student who was caring for this patient following surgery. Despite a written hospital policy that nursing students were to work under close and direct supervision of a licensed registered nurse, the court felt the nursing student had a duty to refuse independent care of this complex patient. Because faculty have a duty to allow only competent students the right to practice in the clinical setting, the faculty member in charge should not have assigned this patient to a student who did not have the knowledge and skills needed to safely care for complex patients.

If faculty assign patients to students who are not competent to safely care for their patients, they may be held liable. *Dustin v. DHCI Home Health Services Inc.* (1966) illustrates this point. A male student was given a clinical assignment by his instructor in the emergency department of an acute medical center. The student, who was not aware of universal precautions or the patient's diagnosis of AIDS, was asked to restrain this violent patient. While the patient was being restrained, blood and saliva from the patient's lacerated lip projected into the student's eyes and mouth. The student later tested positive for HIV and filed suit against the school and hospital. The courts upheld the student's right to sue because the student's training in universal bloodborne pathogen precautions and restraint techniques was inadequate, and he should not have been placed in the emergency department. This case emphasizes the duty of nursing programs to adequately supervise and teach their students as well as to ensure that students have the knowledge and skills needed to practice safely (Guido, 2006, p. 206).

Another area of faculty liability focuses on faculty's failure to protect student safety. The case of *Mastrangelo v. West Side Union High School* (1935) applied the concept of negligence to an educational setting and found that educators had a duty to prevent injury to students. However, the charge of liability on the part of the faculty was denied because students were properly instructed on ways to safely handle chemicals, and the school met the requirements for proper warnings about use of the equipment. Although this case did not involve a nursing environment, learning laboratories in nursing programs may pose injury to students. A similar case, *Niles v. Board of Regents of University System of Georgia* (1996), involved a doctoral chemistry student who suffered an injury following an explosion. The court accepted the position of the university because the student was legally required to be responsible for his own safety.

Nursing students also receive extensive instruction on safety measures to follow when administering nursing care. This knowledge of safety is provided to protect the patient and student from injury. Because faculty have the responsibility to protect students from injury, as clinical educators, diligence must be applied when assessing students' learning environments in an attempt to determine the potential for student injury. As educators we have the responsibility to fully inform our students of the dangers inherent in the learning environment and take reasonable steps to prevent them from occurring (Goudreau & Chasens, 2002). Personal safety should be emphasized during the first weeks of nursing school and throughout the program. For this reason, many nursing programs do not allow students to enter the clinical environment until they have spent time in clinical laboratories with instructor-supervised practice sessions on safety concepts. As nurse educators we have a duty to protect our students from injury in the same manner as we protect our patients from injury. Students are also responsible for their own safety in the clinical environment and must ask for help when needed before placing themselves in a dangerous situation.

When students conduct themselves in an unsafe manner in the clinical setting, the lives and welfare of patients assigned to them may be jeopardized. It is imperative that faculty adhere to the well-defined policies that ensure the due process rights of these students. Misconduct by students is categorized as either disciplinary or academic. Disciplinary misconduct involves a student's failure to comply with the school's code of conduct or rules and regulations; examples include cheating, plagiarism, and unethical behavior. Academic misconduct in nursing education involves a student's grades or unsafe clinical performance. In lawsuits involving dismissals due to academic misconduct, courts have been reluctant to provide students with protection because they fear judicial intervention will jeopardize professional autonomy and integrity (Lallo, 1992). Courts have primarily assumed a laissez-faire attitude toward academic misconduct cases unless arbitrary or capricious behavior by faculty was demonstrated. Arbitrary or capricious behavior by faculty occurs when faculty fail to follow due process procedures. Due process rights for academic misconduct require that students be adequately notified about their academic performance, including deficiencies that need to be improved within certain time frames to allow students' continuation in an educational program (Spink, 1983). Faculty who fail to protect students' due process rights in cases of academic misconduct risk litigation.

Osinski (2003) reviews cases involving nursing students' academic misconduct and faculty adherence to due process rights of students. These cases may help you to understand your responsibility as a clinical educator to ensure your clinical nursing students maintain their due process rights in situations of academic misconduct. In the case of *Gaspar v. Bruton* (1975), a nursing student was dismissed from the nursing program for unsatisfactory clinical performance. The student had completed more than two thirds of the nursing program, was on probation for two months, and was informed that she would be dismissed if her clinical deficiencies did not improve. When her clinical performance did not improve, she was told that she was being dismissed. She was offered a second conference to question the evidence supporting the faculty's decision for dismissal as well as to present evidence in her own defense. The courts ruled that the student had been afforded greater due process consideration than usually is required in academic dismissal. Faculty satisfied their due process responsibilities by informing the student of her impending failure and giving the student time to improve her clinical performance.

A similar case, *University of Missouri v. Horowitz* (1978), involved a medical student who was dismissed for a clinical failure. The student had been offered remedial help and had several conferences with faculty to help her improve. The defendant claimed she had not been given the opportunity to meet with the committee that made the final decision. The Court of Appeals ruled that the student should have been afforded full due process including a hearing with the committee that made the final decision. However, the decision was overturned by the Supreme Court, which ruled that the student was afforded more than adequate due process.

A case in 1987, *Clements v. Hassau County*, featured a nursing student who was dismissed from the program in her last year at a community college for "unsafe clinical behavior" and "failure to maintain cleanliness." After she exhausted the college's grievance procedure for grade dispute, the faculty decision was upheld. The student filed a suit claiming the faculty prevented her graduation. The U.S. Court of Appeals would not intervene unless bad faith or ill will was demonstrated, so it refused to overturn the faculty decision (Parrott, 1993, p. 16). In an earlier, yet similar case in 1986, *Morin v. Cleveland Metro General Hospital*, another nursing student was dismissed during her senior year for unsafe clinical practice. The student appealed the faculty decision, alleging arbitrary and capricious decision making on the part of faculty. However, the administration's committee upheld the faculty's decision. The student filed a suit claiming the instructor was "hostile" toward her and her dismissal was "arbitrary and capricious." The university's decision was upheld (Parrott, 1993, p. 17).

After reviewing these cases, you may realize that it is often difficult to predict the outcomes of litigation cases involving the care patients received when student nurses, clinical faculty, and healthcare agencies are involved. However, clinical faculty may limit their liability by meeting their responsibilities to students presented extensively in this book.

SUMMARY

This chapter provided an overview of the legal issues related to student performance in the clinical environment and faculty responsibilities for protecting the due process rights of students who may be at risk for failure. Clinical faculty need to understand and follow the criteria established for due process if they want to avoid liability in their roles as clinical educators.

Fear of legal action often weighs heavy on the minds of clinical educators, and for this reason they may hesitate to fail a student who performs poorly in the clinical setting. However, as Johnson (2012) reminds us, "Federal and state courts have frequently upheld the responsibility and right of faculty to evaluate students' clinical performance and dismiss students who have failed to meet the criteria for a satisfactory performance" (p. 43). Novice clinical educators have difficulty evaluating students and failing them for unsafe behaviors because they are unsure about the legitimacy of their judgments and their own understanding of how students are expected to practice in clinical settings (Scanlan, 1996; Wall, 1998). We hope that this book will help alleviate your fears as a clinical educator who needs to make those difficult decisions about nursing students' clinical competencies.

Regardless of their fears and uncertainties, clinical faculty must ensure learning experiences for students that provide them with opportunities to develop the knowledge, skills, and abilities needed to become competent practitioners. Faculty are expected to make judgments and decisions about their students' abilities to satisfactorily meet clinical objectives and core competencies. Finally, if students are unable to practice safely in the clinical environment, faculty have the legal and ethical responsibility to deny academic progression in the nursing program.

CASE STUDIES

1. During the semester, a student received information about the safety requirements for tube feeding administration and was validated on the procedure in the laboratory setting. While at the clinical site, you assigned this second-year student to a patient who was to receive a 10 a.m. feeding via a nasogastric tube. You instructed the student to gather the equipment she would need and to come get you when she was ready to do the procedure. Before entering the patient's room, you asked the student about the safety measures she would

follow before beginning the tube feeding. The student did not state "check for nasogastric tube placement before giving the feeding" and explain how this would be done.

   a. How should faculty react to this initial event of clinical unpreparedness?

   b. What responsibility do faculty have when they first discover a student is unprepared to care for a given patient in the clinical setting?

   c. What responsibilities do students have for their continual learning?

   d. If this student continues to jeopardize patient safety when caring for assigned patients, what is your responsibility as a clinical instructor? How would you handle this type of situation?

2. A third-year nursing student took a 7½-hour-old infant from the nursey to be breastfed by his mother. The student misread the infant's armband and gave the newborn to the wrong mother. The error was discovered a few minutes later, and the infant was returned to the nursery by one of the registered nurses. The infant's mother did not witness the event, but was informed later by the staff nurse who had returned the infant to the nursery. No harm occurred, and the mother and infant were discharged the next day. The mother brought a lawsuit on her behalf and on behalf of the infant for negligence against the nursing student, her instructor, and the hospital. The trial court dismissed the lawsuit as unfounded, and the mother appealed (Guido, 2006).

   a. What is the standard of care owed to this new mother by the nursing student?

   b. Do the actions of the nursing student constitute negligence? Why?

   c. If liability is found against the nursing student, how would you expect the court to rule regarding the potential liability of the student's nursing faculty and the clinical agency? Explain you answer.

   d. How would you decide this case?

REFERENCES

Aiken, T. D. (2004). *Legal, ethical and political issues in nursing* (2nd ed.). Philadelphia, PA: F. A. Davis.

Blanding v. Richland Memorial Hospital, No. JR 155725 (1988). *Medical Malpractice Verdicts, Settlements and Experts, 4*(5), 22.

Brent, N. J. (2004a). The law and the nurse educator: A look at legal cases. In L. Caputi & L. Englemann (Eds.), *Teaching nursing: The art and science* (pp. 813–846). Glen Ellyn, IL: College of DuPage Press.

Brent, N. J. (2004b). The law and nursing students: Answers you will want to know. In L. Caputi & L. Englemann (Eds.), *Teaching nursing: The art and science* (pp. 847–860). Glen Ellyn, IL: College of DuPage Press.

Clements v. County of Nassau, 835 F.2d 1000 (2nd Cir. 1987).

Davis, S. H. (2002). Glossary of legal terms. *Plastic Surgical Nursing, 22*(4), 188–193.

Dimora v. Cleveland Clinic Foundation, 683 N.E.2d 1175 (Ohio App. 1996).

Dustin v. DHCI Home Health Services, Inc., 673 So.2d 356 (La App. 1996).

Emerson, R. J. (2007). Legal and ethical implications in the clinical education setting. In *Nursing education in the clinical setting* (pp. 86–101). St. Louis, MO: Mosby Elsevier.

Gaberson, K. B., & Oermann, M. H. (2015). Ethical and legal issues in clinical teaching. In *Clinical teaching strategies in nursing* (4th ed., pp. 89–112). New York, NY: Springer.

Gasper v. Bruton, 513 F.2d 843 (Okla. App 1975).

Glasgow, M, E. S., Dreher, H. M., & Oxholm, C. (2012). *Legal issues confronting today's nursing faculty.* Philadelphia; PA: F. A. Davis.

Goudreau, K. A., & Chasens, E. R. (2002). Negligence in nursing education. *Nurse Educator, 27*(1), 42–46.

Guido, G. W. (2006). Academic settings. In *Legal and ethical issues in nursing* (4th ed., pp. 495–513). Upper Saddle River, NJ: Pearson/Prentice Hall.

Humpert v. Bay Medical Center, WL 22442923 (Mich. App. October 28, 2003).

Johnson, E. G. (2012). The academic performance of students: Legal and ethical issues. In D. M. Billings & J. A. Halstead (Eds.), *Teaching in nursing: A guide for faculty* (4th ed., pp. 33–52). St. Louis, MO: Elsevier/Saunders.

Lallo, D. (1992).Student challenges to grades and academic dismissal: Are they losing battles? *Journal of College and University Law, 18*, 577–593.

Lewallen, L. P., DeBrew, J. K., & Stump, M. R. (2014). Regulations and accreditation requirements for preceptors' use in undergraduate education. *Journal of Continuing Education in Nursing, 45*(9), 1–4.

Lovett v. Lorain Community Hospital, No. 03CA00083000 (Ohio Ct. App. Feb. 11, 2004).

Mastrangelo v. West Side Union High School, 2 Cal 2d, 540 (1935).

Miller, D. (1996). *Social justice*. Oxford, UK: Clarendon.

Morin v. Cleveland Metro General Hospital, 516 N.E. 2d 257 (Ohio, 1986).

Niles v. Board of Regents of University System of Georgia, 473 SE2d, 735, Ga 328 (1996).

O'Conner, A. B. (2006). Ethical and legal issues in nursing education. In *Clinical instruction and evaluation: A teaching resource* (2nd ed., pp. 293–312). Sudbury, MA: Jones and Bartlett.

Osinski, K. (2003). Due process rights of students in cases of misconduct. *Journal of Nursing Education, 42*(2), 55–58.

Parrott, T. (1993). Dismissal for clinical deficiencies. *Nurse Educator, 18*(6), 14–17.

Patton, C. W., & Lewallen, L. P. (2015). Legal issues in clinical nursing education. *Nurse Educator, 40*(3), 124–128.

Rottenstein Law Group. (n.d.). What is procedural due process? Retrieved from http://www.rotlaw .com/legal-library/what-is-procedural-due-process/

Scanlan, J. M. (1996). *Clinical teaching: The development of expertise.* Doctoral dissertation, University of Manitoba, Canada.

Scanlan, J. M. (2001). Dealing with the unsafe student in clinical practice. *Nurse Educator, 26*(1), 23–27.

Shipman, B. (2010). The role of communication in the patient–physician relationship. *Journal of Legal Medicine, 31*(4), 433–442.

Southeastern Oklahoma State University, Master of Arts in Clinical Mental Health Counseling. (n.d.). Due process (appeals). Retrieved from http://homepages.se.edu/cmhc/admission /due-process-appeals/

Spink, L. (1983). Due process in academic dismissals. *Journal of Nursing Education, 22*, 305–306.

The Free Dictionary. (n.d.). Due process of law. Retrieved from http://legal-dictionary.thefreedictionary.com/Due+Process+of+Law

University of Missouri v. Horowitz, 435 U.S. 78 (1978), No. 76-695.

Wall, K. (1998). *The use of intuition by expert clinical nursing teachers in the assessment of the clinical performance of students.* Master's thesis, University of Manitoba, Canada.

Trends in Technology

CHAPTER 12

Integrating Technology into Classroom and Clinical Education

OBJECTIVES

- Identify a variety of technological resources that can be integrated into nursing education.
- Discuss considerations regarding integrating technological choices into the curriculum.
- Devise strategies for the successful integration of technology into the classroom.

With the advance of technology in every aspect of life, nurse educators will be hard-pressed to find a nursing program that has not yet integrated some sort of technology into their curriculum. The challenge for new faculty is not whether there will be technology, but rather which technology to adopt and how best to integrate this pedagogy into the curriculum. The educator must be mindful of the many choices of technological resources on the market, because he or she is the one who ultimately will decide which is most applicable for a specific teaching/learning experience.

Some general considerations need to be taken into account when determining the most appropriate technology to integrate into specific courses. Although there is no consensus as to which technology is best, the instructor should consider the type of resource, students' learning styles, teaching preferences, availability of support, ease of use, applicability to the program, pedagogical soundness, ease of integration, and effectiveness in evaluating outcomes.

Faculty may want to pay close attention to their own skills and their ability to use these instructional tools effectively to implement teaching strategies, monitor the level of student engagement, and measure student learning outcomes. We do not suggest that technology should be integrated into a course just because it exists; however, if you intend to use a certain technology, it is important to consider the type of support that exists to aid the implementation, whether there are processes in place to guide the selection of appropriate resources, and whether methodology is available to assess the effectiveness of the technology.

Too many technologies integrated into any one course can lead to students being overwhelmed and the desired learning outcomes not being met. Choose the technology that you can use to enhance your course and that matches best with your teaching style. Remember, technology does not replace the teacher; it is only a tool the teacher can use.

This chapter introduces and describes several technological resources that have been successfully integrated into nursing programs. The list is in no way exhaustive; however, it forms a starting point for new faculty. The benefits and challenges of these resources are presented in a table at the end of the chapter. Web addresses are also included to make it easy to access some of the technology sites.

The following are some commonly used technological resources:

- Social media
- Clinical simulation
- Online teaching/learning platforms such as Moodle and Blackboard
- Massive open online courses (MOOCs)
- Telehealth
- Faculty lecture presentation methods such as Camtasia Studio and Adobe Connect
- Assistive technological devices
- Technology use in clinical settings
- Digitalized classrooms: tablets, electronic screens, interactive smartboards, and data projections
- Digital resources: iPads, student response systems (SRSs)

SOCIAL MEDIA

Touminen, Stolt, and Salminen (2014) define social media as "information networks and information technology that utilizes a form of communication dealing with interactive and user-generated content and creating and maintaining relationships between people." Examples of social media include blogs, wikis, Twitter, emails, YouTube, Instagram, and Facebook. These types of technologies are regarded as student centered. They encourage rapid communication between students and other students as well as between students and faculty. Students and faculty are challenged to be current in their thinking and creative in their approach to education. These types of technology are also regarded as time- and cost-effective ways to deliver education. Social media is, in most cases, free and easy to access, and it encourages students' engagement and participation.

Mizra (2014) suggests the following strategies for faculty who are planning to incorporate social media into the classroom:

- Start by setting a good example. Be prepared, be consistent, and be flexible.
- Create a Facebook page for the class and manage it regularly.
- Develop a Twitter channel and require all students to follow you.
- When possible, use Skype or other such media for guest speakers.
- Use Adobe Connect to carry out lectures.

Although less commonly used in some nursing programs, the technologies listed in **Table 12-1** may be great choices for educators.

TABLE 12-1 Less-Well-Known Technology	
Technology	**Uses**
• Edmondo	Classes meet online. Send emails and messages to students. Add extra resources for students.
• Edublogs • Planboard	Create a live online learning community. Provide instant response/feedback. Create a classwork calendar to share with students.
• Capzles	Use to illustrate reports.
• Lore	Social media site for educational purposes.
• Study Blue	Mobile app for uploading educational material.
• Camtasia	Create voiceover lectures.
• Lesson Cast	Use for teacher-to-teacher communication.
• Live Binders	Online way to organize and share binders.
• Knewton	Student tracking system.
• Virtual World	Online environment occupied by avatars.
• Second Life	Online platform for education delivery (http://secondlife.com).

Data from TeachThought. (2013). 15 examples of new technology in education. Retrieved from http://www.teachthought.com/technology/15-examples-of-new-technology/

SIMULATION

It is highly likely that as a new faculty member you will be using simulations in the nursing program. Simulation in nursing education is a concept that has been in existence for many decades. More recently, clinical simulation has rapidly expanded to become a well-accepted pedagogical approach to teaching skilled nursing in a laboratory setting using high-, medium-, or low-fidelity manikins and/or human patient simulators (HPSs). Simulation provides students with the opportunity to practice clinical skills in a safe, nonthreatening environment without fear of injuring a patient.

There are several educational theories that support the development and use of simulation as pedagogy. One theory that seems most applicable is that of constructivism (Jeffries, 2014). This theory states that learning is a process of constructing meaning. It is how people make sense of their experiences (Jeffries, 2014). This approach to practice encourages students to synthesize their knowledge in a realistic, nonthreatening environment. The new National League for Nursing (NLN) Jeffries simulation theory (Jeffries, 2015) provides a framework within which to design and implement a simulation experience. It suggests that prior to designing a simulation experience, there should be discussion about the type of equipment, appropriateness of the practice environment, and predetermined participant and facilitator roles.

High-fidelity simulation equipment is designed with systems that generate preprogrammed behaviors such as coughing, apnea, hypertension, or tachycardia. The instructor has predesigned clinical scenarios that prompt behaviors from the simulator; students are then expected to react to these responses as if caring for a live patient using high-level critical thinking. In simulation, learning outcomes are achieved when the educational methodology is student focused rather than teacher focused. The simulation experience encourages the student to think critically and to construct meaning from the experience based on the learner's own knowledge and prior experiences. Immediately following the simulation activity there is a mandatory period of debriefing in which students have the opportunity to reflect on all aspects of the experience.

Debriefing is acknowledged as an integral part of the simulation experience. If the simulation was videotaped, it is played back for students to watch their performance. During the debriefing the teacher acts as a guide or mentor to facilitate student learning, pointing out what was carried out appropriately and what was not. Skilled debriefing is a practiced art that the simulation leader will become more familiar with as he or she repeats the technique.

The benefits of clinical simulation have been widely discussed and reported in the nursing literature. Valler-Jones (2014) emphasizes that simulation in education has been found to be a widely accepted approach to training. The benefits and challenges of simulation are listed in **Table 12-2**. Worth mentioning is that students report that simulation training has left them with feelings of empowerment, independence, and confidence in their skills.

TABLE 12-2 Benefits and Challenges of Some Current Technologies

Technology Type	Uses	Benefits	Challenges
Social media: Prezi, SlideRocket, SlideShare, Vimeo, and Voki	Communication Group projects Research Information management	Encourage good communication skills Require educators to be innovative and to engage in new pedagogies Provide cost- and time-effective nursing education	Provide opportunities for ethics violations Issue of confidentially Privacy issues Potential violation of Health Insurance Portability and Accountability Act (HIPAA) laws
Social networking sites: Google, Google Plus, LinkedIn, Twitter, Second Life, Facebook E-folio creation sites: Google Googlios and Wordpress Literature management software: Mendeley	Store and share information	Free (in most cases), easy to use, and offer the opportunity to strengthen learning, participation, communication, and engagement Enable students to work independently, yet allow for networks to form between students Provide new technological innovations Applicable to students of differing learning styles Increase faculty learning opportunities Facilitate distance learning Provide opportunities for research Student familiarity Address several learning styles Allow for innovative group projects	Lack of adequate support and resources in some programs Can be costly to integrate and sustain Some teachers and students fear new technology Rapid evolution of technologies can result in students and faculty unfamiliarity with what is current

(continued)

TABLE 12-2 Benefits and Challenges of Some Current Technologies (*continued*)

Technology Type	Uses	Benefits	Challenges
Online teaching/learning systems: Moodle, Blackboard, MOOCs	Teaching Communication Resources such as study guides Syllabi Texts Testing Evaluation	Promote constructivist model of education and encourage more individualized student communication Increase accessibility for students in rural areas and for those whose responsibilities prohibit them from attending traditional face-to-face classes Increase collaboration between nursing students and colleagues in other geographic areas Promote group activities, thereby increasing opportunities for social professionalism Promote interdisciplinary teams through participation in online videoconferencing, group discussion threads, and group chats Facilitate research With proper design, can be more cost-effective than traditional courses with comparable or accelerated levels of learning (Schell & Janicki, 2013) Allow group discussions and group chats Provide students with their grades and immediate feedback	System/technology failures can disrupt learning. Opportunities for plagiarism Lack of human interaction Student complacency Cost to student MOOCs' lack of a personal touch Lack of face-to-face faculty–student interaction Little ability to role model the practical aspects of nursing

Simulation Virtual worlds	Tailored to individual learning (Hsu et al., 2013)	Students feel intimidated by being constantly watched by the professor
Learning clinical practice in a controlled laboratory environment	Students practice skills in a safe environment, where errors in clinical judgment will not result in harm to living patients	Some students feel angry at having to speak to a "fake patient"
Unfolding case studies	Possibility to practice one or more skills in specific situations	Students can be anxious at times because the scenarios can appear quite real
Formative evaluation	Students learn the importance of prioritizing nursing care interventions	Costly to initiate and support
Summative evaluation	Opportunities to practice physical assessment skills until mastery is achieved	Faculty and students need to have great communication skills
High-stakes assessment	Prepare the student for real-life situations	Need for extensive faculty training and preparation to run the simulation
	Instructor able to provide more personalized attention to each student	Limited research to demonstrate effectiveness (Hsu et al., 2013)
	Debriefing after each scenario provides students with opportunities to review and learn more about what they just experienced	
	Students feel empowered	
	Students able to practice independently at a faster rate when they enter the ward	
	Students report feeling competent in clinical skills	
	Great opportunity for faculty to immediately assess student skills	
	Can be used as an orientation and training tool for new employees to establish a base of expectations	
	Applicable to the constructivist theory of learning (Cook, 2012)	

(continued)

TABLE 12-2 Benefits and Challenges of Some Current Technologies (*continued*)

Technology Type	Uses	Benefits	Challenges
Telehealth	Delivery of health care from a distance through electronic information and telecommunication Done through video conferencing, online health information, email, and online communication with healthcare providers Electronic health records Video or online doctor visits	Delivery of nursing care without the hindrance or barrier of time and distance Patients and families have increased access to care Easier access to care by lower socioeconomic-level patients and those who have chronic illnesses Lower healthcare costs for patients and the healthcare system Improved health outcomes Higher quality of care and quality of life for patients Increased social support for patients, their families, and healthcare providers Increased education opportunities for healthcare providers Remote monitoring of vital signs, such as blood pressure, or symptoms Timely and effective healthcare delivery	Low contact for patients who prefer face-to-face meetings with their healthcare provider Lack of social interaction for patients who are unable to leave their homes due to mobility issues and who look forward to their provider visit
Wireless technology tools: Laptop computers, smartphones, personal digital assistants (PDAs)	Teaching Communication Research	Average students score higher on tests Encourage innovative teaching strategies Increased student engagement and group activities Increase in student confidence Reduced student anxiety Regular use of technology improves the level of student comfort and satisfaction in using technology	Cost Privacy issues HIPAA issues

		Increased student motivation to learn When integrated appropriately, students have a positive learning experience and so become more involved in classroom activities Promote increased student interactions among students and instructors	
Student response system (SRS)	Voiceover in conjunction with PowerPoint lectures Web conferencing with students Classroom assessment	Students can review at their own time and pace No limit on time and place Convenient for students and faculty Live interaction between students and faculty Great opportunities for group discussion Presented via commonly used Adobe Flash Player technology Allows for entire class assessment Immediate feedback Teacher can clarify misunderstandings Students tend to be more connected with the material being taught	Time it takes faculty to create the voiceover Technology failure Prohibitive cost Student must have access to a computer Designated time for meeting may not be convenient to all Can be cost prohibitive Some students may be intimidated by the technology

Simulation is being used not only as an adjunct to clinical education, but also in a variety of other settings such as orientation for new staff, assessing skills competencies for continuing education, staff development training, certification training, skills training, and interdisciplinary communication. Additionally, according to Aebersold and Tschannen (2013), simulation has been demonstrated to be an effective method for training practicing nurses for new procedures, communication processes, and both skill-based and non–skill-based techniques. These types of training can be done using a variety of methodologies, ranging from simple role play to the use of high-fidelity and virtual simulators.

Critical to the appropriate use of simulation is the training for the healthcare faculty member. Although it is known that simulation is more about the educational methodology than the skilled use of the technology, anyone responsible for any aspect of simulation integration has a responsibility to be trained in the use of the resources as well as the pedagogical approach to this type of clinical practice. Additionally, successful integration of simulation into the curriculum as a pedagogical approach will rely on the full support of employers (i.e., the university or college administration).

Simulation can be used for a series of unfolding case studies. It is very effective for use in faculty development, formative and summative evaluation, and high-stakes assessment (Jeffries, 2014).

ONLINE TEACHING AND LEARNING SYSTEMS

Online instructional systems have become second nature in many nursing programs. Often online teaching systems are used to deliver education either fully online or in a hybrid format. A course is regarded as being fully online when 80 percent of the course content is offered online. When 30–79 percent of the content is delivered online, the course is regarded as blended or hybrid. When less than 30 percent of the course is offered online, it is regarded as being a face-to-face (F2F) class.

The Online Learning Consortium (OLC), previously known as the Sloan Consortium, is an organization that provides training programs for online instructors, including training on the development of rubrics for assessing the effectiveness of online courses. More information about this organization and its role in promoting and evaluating online education throughout the country can be obtained online at http://olc.onlinelearningconsortium.org/effective_practices/assessing-effectiveness -online-educator-preparation.

The OLC's goal is to support institutions as they develop online teaching goals and to provide a framework to assist these institutions in meeting their goals. The premise of the OLC is based on the five pillars of quality of online education—access, learning effectiveness, teacher satisfaction, student satisfaction, and scale (institution commitment to achieving capacity versus cost-effectiveness).

New faculty unfamiliar with online pedagogy are advised to spend time learning this approach before delving into this method of teaching. Graduate programs, in particular, have focused on providing synchronous and asynchronous levels of education. This type of teaching increases accessibility for students who may be in distant and remote locations or who have other responsibilities that prevent them from attending F2F classes.

Teaching/Learning Platforms

During orientation to a new faculty position and/or staff development role, employers provide opportunities for incoming employees to become familiar with the online learning system that is in place. Faculty who have no previous online teaching experience will no doubt require extensive training in using the system as well as in converting their courses to the online mode. Several platforms are available; however, this text will focus on two of the most commonly used ones—Moodle (www.moodle.com) and Blackboard (www.blackboard.com).

According to Thiele et al. (2014), Moodle is one of the most predominant technologies adopted by colleges and nursing programs. Moodle provides a comprehensive way to present all aspects of teaching and communication. Students can not only access all teaching/learning material, but also communicate with their professors and classmates at the same time. Students can also be tested remotely at any time of the day or night, no matter where they live in the world.

Blackboard is another learning management system that is often used in many colleges and universities. It provides a system for course delivery and course management. Students' progress can be tracked, and their success in the course analyzed.

There are benefits and challenges to using each of these learning systems, which the teacher must be aware of (see **Table 12-2**). Teachers are obliged to monitor the site frequently to determine student engagement and the effectiveness of learning outcomes. Testing via the Moodle platform is a convenient way to test students; however, there is also a danger of students finding ways to plagiarize while being tested. One of the ways colleges are combating this is by having students log into Moodle with computers that have video monitoring capabilities (Thiele et al., 2014). Monitoring the students limits the possibility of them collaborating with other students or using other resources. Some schools have students report to campus, where they can be monitored during test taking.

MASSIVE OPEN ONLINE COURSES (MOOCs)

In this approach to education, a large number of students in different locations can be taught online with a minimum number of faculty. Touted as the future of nursing education, Skiba (2013) believes MOOCs are one of the answers to the nurse faculty shortage and ultimately the nursing shortage. Implementing online courses provides the teacher with the opportunity to flip the classroom (Hawks, 2014). (See Chapter 4.) Flipping the classroom encourages more active learning as students become more engaged in the learning process. Most of the learning is done outside of the classroom, leaving class time for discussion, clarification, and interaction. A major advantage of this type of delivery is that the teacher is able to reach a larger audience of students located in various sites. Students who are exposed to MOOCs in their studies are more likely to continue with lifelong learning, according to Skiba (2013).

TELEHEALTH

Telehealth, also referred to as telemedicine, is a way of delivering health care from a distance through technology. The U.S. Department of Health and Human Services (2012) defines telehealth as "the use of electronic information and telecommunications to support long distance clinical health care, patient and professional health-related education, public health and health administration." This is done through video conferencing and other technological means. Major tenets of telehealth are the expected decrease in patients' hospital readmission, decrease in healthcare costs, increased access to care, and improved health of the population. Patients, families, healthcare providers, and the healthcare system are all impacted by telehealth.

Telehealth is particularly applicable to rural and underserved communities. Care may be administered via real-time communication with the healthcare provider via telephone or webcam, or by what is known as "store and forward information." In this type of telehealth, information such as images and clinical results are transmitted via live video to a healthcare provider, who stores the data and later forwards the information to an appropriate specialist to interpret and evaluate the patient remotely. Telehealth promises to be a very useful technological approach for nurses administering health care and for nursing students' clinical experiences. There is extensive information about the emerging area of telehealth in the literature. The U.S. Department of Health and Human Services is a rich resource for more information. Benefits and challenges associated with telehealth are summarized in **Table 12-2**.

FACULTY LECTURE WITH TECHNOLOGY

Today's nursing classroom, in keeping current with modern trends, is of necessity "high tech." Classrooms are digitalized with interactive smartboards, electronic screens, data projections, and cameras (see **Box 12-1**). In some classrooms, students sit at individual

> **Box 12-1** Some Technology Resources Found in a Digitalized Classroom
>
> Computers
> Interactive smartboards
> Electronic screens
> Data projections
> Cameras
> Student response systems
> Tablets

computers with Wi-Fi capability for easy access to online searches. In others, students have personal tablets and smartphones. Faculty control the amount of technology they integrate into the course and the way in which they present their course material to students, whether in class or online. Some faculty create learning modules that are uploaded to teaching platforms; others may lecture using programs such as Adobe Connect. In this section we will discuss three commonly integrated technologies in the classroom—student response systems (SRSs) or clickers, Camtasia Studio, and Adobe Connect.

Student Response Systems (SRSs)

Systems exist for teachers to carry out real-time formative evaluation of students' understanding of the material being taught. One common way of doing this is through the use of student response systems (SRSs) or "clickers." The clicker, a small handheld device, is electronically connected to a computer system in the classroom podium from which the teacher is delivering the lecture. Each student is assigned a clicker at the start of the class. At certain points within the lecture, the teacher poses a question regarding the content being taught and asks everyone to respond. The teacher gets immediate feedback and can respond to and clarify any misunderstandings instantaneously. According to Patterson et al. (2010), the teacher can assess the entire group of students for comprehension of the material and adjust the lecture accordingly. Students report feeling more connected with what is happening in the classroom, and as such they become more engaged.

Camtasia Studio

Faculty can use Camtasia Studio (www.camtasia.com) to create learning modules and provide voiceover in conjunction with their PowerPoint lectures. The material is uploaded to the web, and students are provided with a link with which to access the material. Students who are unable to attend classes or who need to review the taught material are able to listen to the lectures remotely on their own time and at their own pace, rewinding and replaying as needed. This program works with the commonly used Adobe Flash Player. Students are unable to edit the PowerPoint file, so the educational integrity of the material is protected (Thiele et al., 2014). The main challenge to this technology is the cost, which can be prohibitive.

Adobe Connect

Adobe Connect is a software program used for web conferencing, among other things. Faculty are able to create a webinar or arrange a meeting with all students for lecture or general chat sessions or discussions. To participate, students log into their computers using Adobe Flash Player. More information on this system can be obtained by going to www.adobe.com.

ASSISTIVE TECHNOLOGICAL DEVICES

Students with special technological needs are often overlooked or forgotten in the classroom. Faculty need to remember that there are several assistive technological devices designed for students and faculty with an impairment. Some of these devices are designed to help students with time management, note taking, organization, and much more. Devices range from low to high technology (Coleman, 2011), and may include some of the items listed in **Box 12-2**. Unfortunately, not all faculty have been exposed to students who need these devices, and therefore may not be familiar with their proper use.

Box 12-2 Assistive Technological Devices

- Hearing aids and amplification devices
- Braille note-taking devices and voice recognition devices
- Low-technology items such as pencil grips
- Calculators
- Handheld spell checkers
- Computers with assistive software
- Timer

Reproduced from Renaldo, M., Vanbergeijk, E., & Vlasak, E. (2013). Using apps to aid at school, home, and transitioning to post-secondary environments. *Exceptional Parent, 43*(9), 50–53.

TECHNOLOGY USE IN CLINICAL SETTINGS

Using technological assistance in the clinical setting has become very commonplace. One of the roles of the clinical nurse is to access the patient's electronic medical record (EMR) to obtain information to effectively care for the patient. The nurse is also expected to be competent in using available technology in delivering care. In some organizations, permission to access patient records is granted only to the nursing faculty who accompany students to the clinical site. The faculty will access the patient data and then be responsible for sharing the information with the students.

Faculty not only are expected to become familiar with the EMR, but also must become skilled in the use of the high-tech equipment used to care for patients, must be able to instruct their students on the proper usage, and must explain patient safety considerations during the usage. To accomplish all of this, faculty need to be oriented on the clinical unit prior to taking students there. Arrangements for this level of orientation can be done through the unit manager.

Faculty teaching in different clinical sites have an ethical responsibility to become familiar with the types of equipment used in each of the sites, especially because they may vary from hospital to hospital and even from unit to unit. Remember that students are not permitted to operate equipment that they have not been oriented to and signed off on as being competent in using.

In addition to patient equipment, some organizations permit students to use personal handheld computers, personal digital assistants (PDAs), electronic physician's desk references (PDRs), tablets, and other patient data collection equipment. Be aware that some organizations permit the use of specific personal instruments while denying the use of others. It is the responsibility of the clinical faculty to instruct the students on proper usage of all the types of technology that they will be using in the clinical site.

CASE STUDIES

1. You are the faculty for the first baccalaureate nursing course and want to begin integrating technology into the learning process. Select a technological resource and explain how you will integrate its use into your course to facilitate learning.

2. The sophomore nursing course you are teaching uses multiple handouts to reinforce the content. Each semester you need to ensure there are enough handouts for each student in the class. This is very time consuming for you. As an alternative, you decide to use technology to ensure all students have access to the necessary handouts. Select a technological resource that both you and the students can use, and explain how you will integrate its use into your course.

3. You are faculty for the capstone course, which is the final course in the nursing program. Students will soon graduate and take the NCLEX-RN exam. Throughout this course you want to use technology to help the students remediate all prior nursing program content. Which technological resources would you make available to students, and how would you plan for this?

REFERENCES

Aebersold, M., & Tschannen, D. (2013). Simulation in nursing practice: The impact on patient care. *OJIN: The Online Journal of Issues in Nursing, 18*(2), 6.

Coleman, M. B. (2011). Successful implementation of assistive technology to promote access to curriculum and instruction for students with physical disabilities. *Physical Disabilities: Education and Related Services, 30*(2), 2–22.

Cook, M. J. (2012). Design and initial evaluation of a virtual pediatric primary care clinic in Second Life. *Journal of the American Academy of Nurse Practitioners, 24*(9), 521–527.

Hawks, S. (2014). The flipped classroom: Now or never? *AANA Journal, 82*(4), 264–269.

Honeywell HomMed. (2012, July). How telehealth impacts healthcare reform. Telehealth and healthcare reform: A white paper. Retrieved from https://www.honeywelllifecare.com/lifestream-resources/

Hsu, E. B., Li, Y., Bayram, J. D., Levinson, D., Yang, S., & Monahan, C. (2013). State of virtual reality based disaster preparedness and response training. *PLOS Currents, 5.* Retrieved from http://currents.plos .org/disasters/article/state-of-virtual-reality-vr-based-disaster-preparedness-and-response-training

Jeffries, P. (2014). *Clinical simulation in nursing education: Advanced concepts, trends and opportunities.* Philadelphia, PA: Walters Kluwer Health.

Jeffries, P. (2015). *The NLN Jeffries simulation theory.* Philadelphia, PA: Wolters Kluwer Health.

Mizra, S. (2014). How teachers can use social media in the classroom. Phoenix Forward Perspectives. Retrieved from https://globaldigitalcitizen.org/how-teachers-can-use-social-media-in-the-classroom

Patterson, B., Kilpatrick, J., & Woebkenberg, E. (2010). Evidence for teaching practice: The impact of clickers in a large classroom environment. *Nurse Education Today, 30*(7), 603–607. doi:10.1016/j. nedt.2009.12.008

Renaldo, M., Vanbergeijk, E., & Vlasak, E. (2013). Using apps to aid at school, home, and transitioning to post-secondary environments. *Exceptional Parent, 43*(9), 50–53.

Schell, G. P., & Janicki, T. J. (2013) Online course pedagogy and the constructivist learning model. *Journal of the Southern Association for Information Systems, 1*(1). doi: http://dx.doi.org/10.3998/ jsai.11880084.0001.104

Second Life. (2014). Home page. Retrieved from http://secondlife.com

Skiba, D. (2013). MOOCs and the future of nursing. *Nursing Education Perspectives, 34*(1), 202–204.

TeachThought. (2013). 15 examples of new technology in teaching. Retrieved from http://www.teach thought.com/technology/15-examples-of-new-technology/

Thiele, A., Mai, J., & Post, S. (2014). The student-centered classroom of the 21st century: Integrating Web 2.0 applications and other technology to actively engage students. *Journal of Physical Therapy Education, 28*(1), 80–93.

Touminen, R., Stolt, M., & Salminen, L. (2014). Social media in nursing education: The view of the students. *Education Research International, 2014.* doi: http://dx.doi.org/10.1155/2014/929245

U.S. Department of Health and Human Services, Health Resources and Services Administration. (2014). What is telehealth? Retrieved from http://www.hrsa.gov/healthit/toolbox/RuralHealth ITtoolbox/Telehealth/whatistelehealth.html

Valler-Jones, T. (2014). The impact of peer-led simulations on student nurses. *British Journal of Nursing, 23*(6), 321–326.

Links to Some Commonly Used Nursing Technology Resources

RESOURCE	USES
Education and Technology	
Project Muse: http://muse.jhu.edu	Provides digital humanities and social sciences content; journal collections support a wide array of research needs at academic, public, special, and school libraries.
FreeNurseTutor: http://freenursetutor.com	An easy, practical way to add computer-based learning activities to current teaching methods. Activities such as games and Flash & Match help students to study in an interactive way.
Open Educational Resources for Nursing Education: http://nursing.gwu.edu/open-educational-resources-nursing-education	A list of interactive multimedia learning materials that provide scenarios and explanations for the field of nursing.
An Online Exploration of Human Anatomy and Physiology: http://www.getbodysmart.com	Examines the structures and functions of the human body using a series of interactive illustrations.
Understanding Medical Words: A Tutorial from the National Library of Medicine: http://www.nlm.nih.gov/medlineplus/medicalwords.html	Teaches new nursing students the meaning of medical words.
Dimensions of Culture: http://www.dimensionsofculture.com	Assists learners in understanding how to be more effective with patients and families from different cultures.
Websites and Blogs	
Twitter: https://twitter.com	Microblogging social media site where you can send and receive tweets in 140 characters or less. Share links to resources, photos, and videos; follow current events.
WordPress: https://wordpress.com	
Edublogs: http://edublogs.org	
Google Blogger: https://www.blogger.com	
Tumblr: https://www.tumblr.com	

RESOURCE	USES
Free Courses and Course Content	
Merlot: http://www.merlot.org	A curated collection of free and open online teaching, learning, and faculty development services contributed to and used by an international education community.
iTunes U: https://itunes.apple.com/us/genre /itunes-u/id40000000?mt=10	
Khan Academy: https://www.khanacademy .org	
Video	
QuickTime Pro: http://www.apple.com /quicktime/extending/	Record, edit, play, and export videos.
YouTube: https://www.youtube.com	Create a free account to upload your own videos, or search for educational video content.
TeacherTube: http://www.teachertube.com	Free community for sharing instructional videos and content for teachers and students.
Vimeo: https://vimeo.com	Upload your own videos, or search for educational video content.
TED: https://www.ted.com/talks	Over 2100 talks to stir your curiosity.
Presentations	
Prezi: https://prezi.com	Free, web-based presentation application that uses motion, zoom, and other effects to create dynamic presentations.
PowerPoint: https://products.office.com /en-us/powerpoint	Microsoft Office application for creating presentations.
Keynote: http://www.apple.com/mac /keynote/	Apple's application for creating presentations; available for Mac computers.
Assessment	
Qualtrics: https://www.qualtrics.com	Online survey for assessment and research.
Rubistar: http://rubistar.4teachers.org	Tool for creating and editing your own rubrics.
Poll Everywhere: http://www.polleverywhere .com	Tool to create online polls or to gather students' live responses.
CourseNotes: http://www.course-notes.org	Provides access to notes, outlines, vocabulary terms, study guides, and practice exams.
Turnitin: http://www.turnitin.com	An online program used to check students' writing for plagiarism and assist teachers in grading papers; allows for anonymous review of papers.

Index